DR ATKINS

Quick & Easy

NEW DIET

COOKBOOK

Also by Dr Robert C. Atkins

The Vita-Nutrient Solution

DR ATKINS

Quick & Easy

NEW DIET

COOKBOOK

•

Dr Robert C. Atkins

and Veronica Atkins

POCKET BOOKS

London • Sydney • New York • Tokyo • Singapore • Toronto

This edition published by Pocket Books, 2002
An imprint of Simon & Schuster UK Ltd
A Viacom Company

7 9 10 8 6

Simon & Schuster UK Ltd
Africa House
64-78 Kingsway
London WC2B 6AH

www.simonsays.co.uk

Simon & Schuster Australia
Sydney

A CIP catalogue record for this book is available from the British Library

ISBN 0-7434-6241-6

Printed and bound in Great Britain
by Cox & Wyman Ltd, Reading, Berkshire

This publication contains the opinions and ideas of its author. It is intended to provide
helpful and informative material on the subjects addressed in the publication. It is sold
with the understanding that the author and publisher are not engaged in rendering
medical, health, or any other kind of personal professional services in the book. The
reader should consult his or her medical, health or other competent professional before
adopting any of the suggestions in this book or drawing inferences from it. Pregnant
women and people with severe kidney disease are strongly advised not to follow this
diet. The author and publisher specifically disclaim all responsibility for any liability, loss
or risk, personal or otherwise, which is incurred as a consequence, directly or indirectly,
of the use and application of any of the contents of this book.

to my mother, Emma, who would have been very proud of me
—VERONICA ATKINS

• Contents •

Lose Weight, Look Great, and Enjoy Your Food,
by Robert C. Atkins, MD 13

The Best Food You Have Ever Tasted,
by Veronica Atkins 16

WHAT ARE NET CARBS? 18

QUICK & EASY KITCHEN STRATEGIES 19

    CLEAN HOUSE 19

    MANAGING YOUR WEEK 20

    SHOPPING 20

    ORDERING SUPPLIES BY MAIL 20

    EQUIPMENT 21

HIDDEN CARBOHYDRATES 21

HINTS FOR MODIFYING OTHER RECIPES TO THE CONTROLLED CARBOHYDRATE
WAY OF EATING 22

QUICK AND EASY GUIDE TO THE *QUICK & EASY NEW DIET COOKBOOK* 24

Breakfasts 25

    Herbed Scrambled Eggs 27

    Ham and Swiss Cheese Frittata 28

    Creamy Scrambled Eggs with Dill and Smoked Salmon 29

    Baked Eggs in Bacon Rings 30

    Eggs Benedict with Spinach 31

    Carrot and Nut Muffins 32

    Mini Chocolate Chip Muffins 33

    Blueberry Breakfast Scones 34

Hors d'Oeuvre, Appetizers and Snacks 37

    Guacamole 39

    Marinated Goat's Cheese with Oregano 40

    Courgette Rolls with Goat's Cheese 41

    Artichoke Hearts Wrapped in Bacon 42

    Caponata 43

    Baked Goat's Cheese and Ricotta Custards 44

    Devilled Eggs 45

Baked Brie with Sun-Dried Tomatoes and Pine Nuts .. 46

Smoked Salmon Rolls............................. 47

Chicken Liver Pâté with Cloves 48

Salmon-Stuffed Courgettes 49

Soups 51

Cucumber Dill Soup............................. 53

Manhattan Clam Chowder....................... 54

Roasted Pepper Soup............................ 55

French Onion Soup Gratinée 56

Asparagus and Leek Soup 57

Golden Cauliflower-Curry Soup 58

Roasted Vegetable Soup 59

Blue Cheese and Bacon Soup..................... 60

Salads 61

Orange Daikon Salad 63

Fennel Salad with Parmesan 64

Endive Salad with Walnuts and Roquefort 65

Walnut Coleslaw................................ 66

Celeriac Salad 67

Red Cabbage Salad with Feta and Dill............. 68

Greek Salad 69

Mixed Green Salad with Warm Bacon Dressing...... 70

Warm Spinach Salad with Bacon and Pine Nuts 71

Open Sesame Broccoli Salad 72

Salad Niçoise 73

Tri-Colour Salad............................... 74

Shrimp Cocktail with Two Sauces 75

Fresh Greens with Classic Vinaigrette 76

Main Courses 77

EGGS.. 79

Mustard Scrambled Eggs 80

Ricotta and Leek Frittata........................ 81
Smoked Salmon Frittata......................... 82
Herb Kookoo (Frittata with Herbs)............... 83
Egg Salad with Capers 84

SEAFOOD...................................... 85

Scallops with Thyme 86
Thai Coconut-Ginger Shrimp 87
Stir-Fried Prawns with Ginger and Mushrooms 88
Prawn Scampi.................................. 89
Tarragon Prawn Salad 90
Crab and Avocado Salad......................... 91
Sautéed Cod with Lemon-Parsley Sauce 92
Red Snapper with Tomato and Olives 93
Mackerel Fillets with Mustard-Rosemary Mayonnaise. 94
Fish Fillets with Tomatoes and Black Olives 95
Mahi-Mahi with Creole Sauce..................... 96
Oven-Poached Salmon with Dill and Wine 97
Cajun Blackened Tuna 98
Peppers Stuffed with Walnut Tuna Salad 99
Pepper-Crusted Swordfish....................... 100
Squid with Basil and Lime 101

POULTRY 103

Chicken with Lemon and Capers 104
Coconut Chicken Satés with Coriander............ 105
Chicken with Coconut-Plum Sauce 106
Indian Tikka Chicken........................... 107
Chicken with Indian Spices...................... 108
Chicken Paprika............................... 109
Chicken Adobo................................ 110
Chicken Salad with Pesto and Fennel 111
Curried Chicken Salad with Cucumber............ 112
Burgundy Chicken............................. 113
Breast of Duck with Red Wine Sauce.............. 114

PORK 115

Stir-Fried Pork with Water Chestnuts 116
Mustard-Crusted Pork 117
Pork Chops with Orange and Rosemary 118
Pork with Chilli Sauce 119
Peppery Pork Chops............................ 120
Garlic Dill Meatballs 121
Barbecued Spareribs 122

LAMB 123

Grilled Marinated Lamb Chops 124
Grilled Lemon and Rosemary Lamb............... 125
Shortcut Moussaka............................. 126

BEEF 129

Spiced Steak.................................. 130
Filets Mignons with Zesty Wine Sauce............ 131
Rib-eye Steak with Red Wine Sauce.............. 132
Grilled Steaks with Mustard-Herb Rub........... 133
Sirloin Steak with Cognac Mustard Sauce......... 134
Lemon-Thyme Tenderloin with Roasted Vegetables... 135
Beef Burgers with Feta and Tomato 136
Chevapchichi (Spicy Meat Rolls).................. 137
Burrito Beef................................... 138
Chilli Beef Kebabs 139
Burgundy Beef Stew............................ 140
Asian Beef Salad............................... 141

Vegetables 143

Cauliflower with Cumin Seeds................... 144
Grilled Aubergine with Mint Sauce............... 145
Grilled Leeks with Lemon Vinaigrette............. 146
Sautéed Courgettes with Nutmeg 147
Baked Fennel au Gratin 148
Green Beans with Garlic-Tarragon Vinaigrette 149

Mangetout with Hazelnuts 150
Green Beans with Anchovy Sauce 151
Green Bean, Smoked Mozzarella and Tomato Salad... 152
Sprouting Broccoli with Spicy Sausage 153
Green Beans with Sun-Dried Tomatoes
    and Goat's Cheese........................... 154
Sautéed Spinach with Garlic and Olive Oil 155
Puréed Avocado with Garlic and Tarragon 156
Roasted Peppers in Garlic Oil 157
Vegetable Medley.............................. 158
Stir-Fried Vegetables with Mustard Seeds
    and Balsamic Vinegar 159
Stir-Fried Asparagus with Basil 160
Spinach and Cheddar Casserole.................. 161
Sesame Broccoli, Red Pepper and Spinach 162
Tomato-Cucumber Guacamole.................. 163

Sauces....................................... 165

Sorrel Sauce 166
Red Pepper Purée 167
Anchovy Paste................................ 168
Basil Pesto................................... 169
Coriander-Lime Pesto 170
Mint-Cumin Pesto 171
Walnut and Blue Cheese Butter................. 172
Zesty Coriander Butter........................ 173
Peanut Dipping Sauce 174
Cucumber-Dill Sauce 175
Creamy Celery Sauce.......................... 176
Horseradish Cream 177
Caper Tartar Sauce........................... 178
Creamy Mushroom Sauce 179
Quick & Easy Hollandaise 180

Dressings *181*

Quick & Easy Salad Dressing 183
Shallot Orange Vinaigrette 184
Mustard Walnut Vinaigrette 185
Caesar Dressing 186
Smoked Salmon Dressing 187

Breads *189*

Cheddar Cheese Bread 191
Bacon Pepper Bread 192
Sesame Soured Cream Muffins 193
Butter Rum Muffins 194

Desserts *195*

Zabaglione 197
Swedish Cream 198
Coconut Custard Pudding 199
Chocolate Butter Cream 200
Hazelnut Torte 201
Crustless Cheesecake 202
Coconut Cookies 203
Shortcake Veronique with a Kiss of Rum 204
Dr Atkins's Quick & Easy Dessert 205

QUICK & EASY CONTROLLED CARBOHYDRATE FOOD LIST 207
ACKNOWLEDGMENTS 212
ABOUT THE AUTHORS 213

• Lose Weight, Look Great, • and Enjoy Your Food

by Robert C. Atkins, MD

If you're reading this book, you probably have a conflict in your life: you love food – everybody does – yet you need to slim down – and keep the weight off. Moreover, you love not just any food, but mouth-watering, rich and satisfying food. You must feel that you're caught on the horns of a dilemma: the choice between looking and feeling great or eating well.

So will you believe me when I tell you that you *can* have both? Using this very special cookbook, you'll learn to create sumptuous dishes *and* lose weight, all the while making garden-variety (meaning low-fat, calorie-counting) dieters envious. You'll enjoy all the foods that other weight-loss programmes ban. What's more, the recipes in this book have such universal appeal that at a dinner party no one will guess your hidden agenda: that you're simultaneously serving dishes that are helping you control your weight – unless, of course, you choose to share your 'secret' with your guests.

The secret is the Atkins Nutritional Approach™.

Atkins is not just another novelty diet; nor is it simply one of many weight-control options. It's so different from other programmes that if you're new to Atkins you cannot help but say to yourself, 'This is too good to be true!'

However, I'll wager that most of you who have read *Dr Atkins New Diet Revolution* and have been doing Atkins smile when you hear such expressions of disbelief. You know from experience that what I say is true. And those of you new to the Atkins Nutritional Approach™, please understand that it is specifically geared to correct the metabolic imbalance that causes most people to become overweight.

Excess weight – especially a significant amount – may represent an identifiable metabolic disorder called hyperinsulinism. (Of course, being overweight can also simply be the result of consuming excess calories.) A blood test can show if you have it. And if you do, you can correct it – actually, bypass it – by sharply cutting down on your carbohydrate intake. The reason: insulin floods the bloodstream only when excessive amounts of carbohydrate are consumed. So by controlling carbohydrate intake and eating only what we call 'good' carbs and avoiding sugar, refined flour and other nutrient-poor carbs, you can completely manage your insulin problem. As a victim of hyperinsulinism, you are metabolically quite normal, unless and until you eat an excess of refined carbohydrates.

Moderating your carbohydrate intake induces your body to burn primarily fat for energy. After cutting cut back on your carbohydrate intake for 48 hours or more, you will normalize your blood sugar, have more energy and feel much less hungry. Because your hunger is moderated, you'll feel full and satisfied with the food you eat. Yet simultaneously, you're likely to be steadily losing weight. Even better, most people find that they take off inches where they most wanted to rid themselves of unwanted fat.

We now refer to the Atkins Nutritional Approach™ as a controlled carbohydrate approach. While you will be eating low (or lower) carbohydrate foods, the actual amount of carbs you can consume varies greatly. Some people can consume far more than others. Much depends upon how much weight you have to lose, your activity level, age, gender and hormonal status, among other factors. So we feel the term 'controlled', meaning that you monitor your intake of carbohydrates, is more accurate and inclusive. We continue to use the term low carb when referring to foods. By eating low carbohydrate meals, you control your carb intake.

Despite the scientific basis of these controlled carbohydrate principles, we live in an age where the low-fat diet has become the norm and – until now – very few people have questioned it. Restaurants, cookbook authors and dieticians, among others, have tried to convince us that a low-fat diet is, or can be made to be, satisfying. The tide is changing, however. In just the last year, more and more scientific research published in peer-reviewed medical journals has emerged, questioning the science behind the low-fat theory and providing convincing evidence that the controlled carb approach is well grounded in nutritional science. (To review this data, go to www.atkinscenter.com and click on the 'The Science Behind Atkins' section.) This is wonderful news to people like you who are increasingly unhappy with tasteless, unsatisfying food that leaves them hungry a few hours after a meal.

If you have tried to limit fat intake in the mistaken belief that eating less dietary fat will make you slimmer, you've probably found that such food is nowhere near as enjoyable and fulfilling as the food with fat in it. Certainly, that was my experience. At times I have wonder whether the words 'gourmet' and 'masochist' have become synonyms! No matter what other cookbooks claim, fat-free foods taste differently. There is no delicious substitute for butter, heavy cream, pâté, pesto sauce, avocadoes, bacon or steak. Low-fat creations just don't work because fat creates, translates and intensifies flavour; it's what makes you feel sated and full. Your body can't be fooled, nor can your taste buds.

For any weight-loss programme to be successful, it must become a lifetime way of eating. Most diets are doomed to failure because after an individual loses weight, he or she goes back to eating the very same way that initially led to the weight gain. The metabolic imbalance that causes you to become overweight never goes away; instead, you must master it with a permanently changed way of eating. Other weight-control programmes and the cookbooks that promote them expect you to live the rest of your life eating bland, fat-free foods. Those diets fail because the requirements are so stringent and the meals so boring that no one can bear to stay the course.

This book is designed to be your guide to a revolution in eating – what I like to call a new diet revolution. (In truth, this new diet revolution is now forty years old, dating to when I first started recommending it to patients in my medical practice.) Using the recipes in this extraordinary book, you will enjoy cooking and eating real foods. Low carbohydrate gourmet Veronica Atkins, who just happens to be my wife, is the author and her recipes rival those of any restaurant or gourmet magazine. When you taste her creations, you'll become fully aware of just what you have been missing. You'll be clued into a most fascinating paradox: controlling carbohydrates allows you to enjoy meals that are better, richer, and more sumptuous than most everyday foods.

Sitting down to dinner together is precious time for any family, so Veronica has ingeniously created mouth-watering meals that can be prepared quickly. And so the 'Quick & Easy' in the title of this book. That way, you can focus on good food and companionship when enjoying meals with your family and friends. And isn't that what eating should really be about?

• The Best Food You Have Ever Tasted •

by Veronica Atkins

Dr Atkins and I developed this book not only to whet your appetite but also to give you the know-how to lead the controlled carbohydrate lifestyle. We never want you to feel as though you're on a diet, meaning a temporary weight-loss programme that you will abandon once you lose weight. Instead, we want you to enjoy the varied and luxurious cuisine that Atkins offers. Beyond that, we want this to become the way you eat for a lifetime. (Once you've lost weight and achieved your goal weight, you'll be able to consume more healthy carbohydrates but you will still continue to control your carb intake.)

This book is also designed for the busy home cook, so all the recipes can be made in 30 minutes or less. My dishes are easy, flexible, satisfying, substantial, delicious and nutritious. I never skimp on flavours or ingredients. I don't have to, nor would my sentiments about food allow me to do so.

Food has always played a pivotal role in my life. When I was growing up in postwar Europe, food was very scarce, but my family still enjoyed wonderfully creative dishes. As an opera singer, I lived in many countries with unique culinary traditions, which allowed me to discover many new foods and flavours. Then in the United States I met a kindred spirit, a revolutionary doctor, who saw food as something much more powerful than mere sustenance.

My marriage and my work with Dr Atkins and the Atkins Nutritional Approach™ were a natural continuation of my lifelong love affair with food. I began to create low carbohydrate recipes that were easy and delicious. All of our friends would ask me for my secrets. But when doing Atkins, you don't need some secret, complicated way of cooking. Just a few simple steps can start you on a new lifestyle.

You'll be amazed how easy it is to modify your own cooking style to create a low carbohydrate menu. Main-course dishes are wonderfully easy to tailor to Atkins because most of them are already protein-based. The main-dish recipes that follow are some of my favourites. After working with them, you will soon learn how to modify your own favourite main-course recipes to make them perfectly compatible with doing Atkins.

Vegetable dishes are almost as easy to modify. Just keep handy a list of the permissible vegetables and avoid deep-frying or dressing them with carbohydrate-laden sauces based on flour. On the other hand, dressing veggies with butter or olive oil is fine. I have also tried to make the vegetable dishes extra flavourful and luxurious, and so they can often stand on their own as the centerpiece of a meal.

Breads and desserts are a bit harder to modify but not impossible. By testing different substitute ingredients, I have found the best combinations to create delicious lower carbohydrate recipes.

It's important to understand that this book — and the Atkins Nutritional Approach™ itself — isn't about restriction or denial. It is about enjoying food, real food, sumptuous food. I encourage you to explore your palate, try new flavours and see cooking as fun, not a chore. Sadly, the culinary arts have diminished in recent years. Because we are all so pressed for time, prepackaged foods have often taken the place of nutritious home cooking. Such manufactured foods do offer a quick-fix solution to getting dinner on the table, but they are hardly healthy choices. Moreover, people are sick and tired (literally) of the processed so-called foods with little or no fat, no flavour and no pleasure. If you love luxurious foods with rich flavours, there is no other way of eating more suited to rediscovering the joys of home cooking than Atkins. This book will change your perception of cooking and controlling your weight. You will come to view both not as a brief experiment, but a life-long practice; not as an experience to endure, but an ongoing pleasure.

WHAT ARE NET CARBS?

Not all carbohydrates behave the same way in your body. While most carbs — sugar is the best example — are digested and turned into blood sugar (glucose), other carbs behave differently. Some are digested by your body but not turned into glucose and some carbs — such as fibre — are not digested at all and pass through your body as waste. Neither of these types of carbs produces a noted impact on blood sugar levels. You need concern yourself only about the carbs that affect your blood sugar. We call those carbs 'Net Carbs' because they are what remain when you subtract the fibre (and other ingredients such as glycerine and sugar alcohols that may be in reduced carb products). So now our recipes show both the total grams of carbohydrate and the Net Carbs. again, it is only the Net Carbs you need to count in your daily carb count.

QUICK & EASY KITCHEN STRATEGIES

When you cook every day, your kitchen has to be designed to allow you to function quickly and efficiently. Taking control of your pantry and refrigerator makes watching your weight much easier, too. The following practical suggestions should help get your kitchen up and running for the rest of your controlled carbohydrate life:

Clean House

Get rid of temptations! You probably have a lot of refined carbohydrates lurking in your kitchen: sweets, chocolate bars, crackers, crisps, bread crumbs, biscuits, skimmed milk, jams are some of the most obvious culprits. If all members of your household are doing Atkins or you live alone, of course you can get rid of all high carbohydrate temptations. If you can't banish them altogether because it could precipitate a family crisis, do put such foods in a separate part of your pantry and refrigerator. When you are cooking the wonderful dishes in this book, you'll want your shelves instead to be full of the delicious, low carbohydrate ingredients you can use with ease.

If other household members are not doing Atkins with you, you obviously can't toss all those high carb foods. However, if you care about the health of your family, regardless of whether they are overweight or not, do remove the worst offenders: anything made with white flour and trans fats (hydrogenated oils). It's also a good idea to limit children's sugar consumption, both in cereals and such but also in prepared foods and beverages. Getting them in the habit of eating whole-grain breads and cereals now, for example, may help them forestall weight problems later in life. The recipes in this book are appropriate for the whole family, but anyone who chooses to can add a few extra carbohydrates in the form of whole grains, higher carb vegetables or legumes to accompany the main course you've prepared.

Managing Your Week

With a little planning you can create the simple building blocks for your week's dining. If you prepare a few sauces at the start of the week, you can combine them with protein staples (chicken, beef, fish, and so on, see page 207 or a complete list) or leftovers. And you'll end up with a variety of flavourful meals for the whole week. Of course, if you prefer, you can make sauces at the last moment.

For example, if you make Cilantro-Lime Pesto (page 170) you can serve it with grilled chicken the first day, use it in an omelette with feta cheese the following day and then add a tablespoon of it to your tuna salad on another day. So if you make as few as three sauces at the beginning of the week, three meals are practically set.

Shopping

The foundation of the Atkins Nutritional Approach™ is fresh, wholesome ingredients, most of which can be purchased in your supermarket. In fact, shopping for a controlled carbohydrate regimen can make your visits to the supermarket shorter and simpler. In our experience, fresh ingredients are found on the perimeter of the store, where meat, vegetable and dairy sections are located. The store's middle aisles are usually filled with over-processed high carbohydrate foods. Just pass them by. Buy fresh, natural, unprocessed food, and whenever possible, try to find organic foods that are grown without hormones and pesticides. Once a month or so you may need to go to a specialty or health food store for specific ingredients. If you stock up, you'll have what you need for daily use.

Ordering Supplies by Mail

If you cannot find some of the ingredients locally, most are available by mail order and over the Internet. For up-to-date mail-order information on items such as Atkins™ Bake Mix, sugar free syrups, and other Atkins products, go to www.atkinscenter.com.

Equipment

To make quick and easy meals, your kitchen should have certain pieces of the equipment. These few additions to your basic store of pots and pans can greatly reduce both preparation and cooking time.

FOOD PROCESSOR: A must for any kitchen, it allows you to create innumerable dishes and frees you from depending on bottled dressing, sauces and canned soups.

RAMEKINS: Great for baking individual portions, they also reduce cooking time.

OVENPROOF FRYING PAN: Offers the convenience of transferring a dish directly from the stovetop to the oven.

MUFFIN TINS: Reduce the cooling time needed for quick breads.

DOUBLE BOILER: Lets you make delicate sauces or melt cheese.

ENAMEL FRYING PAN: This is Dr Atkins' personal favourite cooking tool.

HIDDEN CARBOHYDRATES

Not that long ago it was hard to figure out the real carbohydrate content and gram count of many foods. But now, with labeling laws in place, the 'carbohydrate grams per serving' is clearly shown in the nutritional description of all processed foods. In assessing carbohydrates, make sure you consider your serving size (usually shown on the top of the label). All too often the serving size, for which carbohydrate grams are measured, is only a small portion of the whole. This can be very misleading, so read all labels carefully. As a rule, when a label states that a portion is 'less than 1 gram' of carbohydrate, you should count it as a full gram because it could be up to 0.99 of a gram. When it comes to counting carbohydrates, it's always better to overestimate.

You may be surprised at some of the foods with high carbohydrate counts. Here are some you should watch out for:

- Luncheon meats, bottled salad dressings, margarine, imitation mayonnaise, ketchup, relish, pickles and diet cheeses. These often have sugars or starches added.

- Prepared gravies and sauces. These often have starches as thickeners or sugars as sweeteners.

- Other carbohydrate-laden sweeteners, such as corn sweetener, corn syrup, corn syrup solids, dextrose, fructose, fruit juice concentrate, glucose, high-fructose corn syrup, honey, invert sugar, lactose, maltose, malt, malt syrup, molasses and raw sugar. Read 'sugar-free' labels carefully. Products may not contain sugar, but they may still have these sweeteners. Also be alert to 'no sugar added' labels because these products may include natural sugars. (A no-sugar added jam will still have the natural sugars from the fruit itself; in small quantities this is not an issue.)

- Dairy products. Remember that, as a rule, the lower the fat content of a milk product, the higher its carbohydrate grams. Use cream, not skimmed milk; use soured cream, not yogurt on the weight loss phases of Atkins.

- Chewing gum, breath mints, cough drops and cough syrups. These often contain sugar and carbohydrates. Be wary.

- 'Low-fat' and 'fat-free' foods. Cutting fat usually means that more sugar has or other sweeterns have been added.

HINTS FOR MODIFYING OTHER RECIPES TO THE ATKINS NUTRITIONAL APPROACH™

- Refer to the Quick & Easy Controlled Carbohydrate Food List in the back of this book (pages 207–9) as a guide to foods you can eat while doing Atkins.

- For dredging, use Atkins™ Bake Mix, soy flour, tofu flour or whey protein instead of flour.

- Use cauliflower, not potatoes, to thicken sauces.

- When onions are cooked, they caramelize, so use minimal amounts, rely on spring onions or add a bit of onion powder instead.

- When a recipe contains several vegetables, refer to the list of Controlled Carbohydrate Vegetables (page 208). Omit any vegetables from the recipe that are not on the list and substitute ones that are. Once you are in the Lifetime Maintenance phase of Atkins, you can be more liberal in your vegetable choices so long as you continue to count carbs.

- Change the ratio of starchy vegetables to meat. In a given recipe, cut back on the amount of starchy vegetables and increase the amount of meat.

- For recipes that call for breading to be sprinkled on top of something, you can try using a mixture of chopped nuts and cheese.

- For spreads and dips, use celery sticks, whole endive leaves, hard-boiled eggs, plain frittatas cut into wedges, pork rinds or whole-grain flatbreads instead of crackers and bread.

- Most baked egg dishes don't need a crust. Just butter your pan well and pour the eggs directly into it.

- Experiment with sugar substitutes. We suggest using a combination of them because when they are mixed together, sweeteners create a synergistic effect. Therefore, less is needed. We recommend not using Equal or aspartame in cooking or baking; they lose their sweetness when heated.*

- Don't assume any food is low in carbohydrate. Read all labels and invest in a carbohydrate gram counter.
  (Or go to www.atkinscenter.com.)

* Although most published scientific studies have proclaimed aspartame (NutraSweet, Equal) to be safe, clinical experience has often indicated otherwise. Headaches, irritability and failure to lose weight or to control blood glucose have all been reported, as well as cross reactions in those who cannot tolerate monosodium glutamate (MSG). Consult your doctor if you have any concern about your use of aspartame. The best advice may be to use it sparingly, preferably blending it with other sweeteners.

QUICK & EASY GUIDE TO
THE QUICK & EASY
NEW DIET COOKBOOK

This cookbook is a companion to *Dr Atkins New Diet Revolution*, which provides an in-depth explanation of the four phases fof the Atkins Nutritional Approach™ and the scientific principles behind it. As you use this cookbook, keep in mind that succeeding on Atkins depends on your accurately counting the total Net Carb grams consumed per day. Each individual has his or her own carbohydrate threshold below which weight loss continues. You should therefore determine how many Net Carbs you have in each meal, and to ensure that you do not exceed your limit, consider any additional carbohydrates you consume in snacks and desserts. We have created recipes in this book that are appropriate to each phase of the Atkins programme. Following are some brief guidelines to keep in mind when choosing a recipe:

During the *Induction Phase*, you should consume no more than 20 grams of carbohydrate a day in the form of salad and other vegetables.

During the *OngoingWeight Loss Phase*, you need to find your own 'Critical Carbohydrate Level', as explained in *Dr Atkins New Diet Revolution*. For the average individual, this level is 30 to 60 grams each day. There are many recipes you can enjoy during these phases; you should wait to make those with more grams Net Carbs or more until you are the later phases.

During the *Pre-maintenance Phase*, you deliberately slow down your weight loss as you slowly increase your daily carbohydrate consumption. Depending on your gender, age, activity level, hormone status and other factors, you may be able to consume as little as 50 grams Net Carbs a day or considerably more.

during the *Lifetime Maintenance Phase*, your goal is simply to maintain your goal weight. You will continue at or slightly above the level you reached in *Pre-maintenance*. We call that your ACE, meaning 'Atkins Carbohydrate Equilibrium', the number of grams of Net Carbs you can consume while neither gaining nor losing weight.

In both the *Pre-maintenance Phase* and the *Lifetime Maintenance Phase*, most people can use all the recipes in this book, including those with the highest Net Carbs per meal and total Net Carb grams per day.

If you find our recipes as useful as we think you will, you will also enjoy the recipes in *Dr Atkins New Diet Revolution*.

Breakfasts

•

Herbed Scrambled Eggs

Ham and Cheese Frittata

Creamy Scrambled Eggs with Dill and Smoked Salmon

Baked Eggs in Bacon Rings

Eggs Benedict with Spinach

Carrot and Nut Muffins

Mini Chocolate Chip Muffins

Breakfast Blueberry Scones

• Herbed Scrambled Eggs •

The delicate flavour of fresh herbs gives scrambled eggs a new dimension. It's really worth the little extra effort.

> NET CARBS* PER SERVING: 2.5 grams
>
> CARBOHYDRATES PER SERVING: 2.5 grams

1 tablespoon butter
6 eggs
2 tablespoons cream
¼ teaspoon salt

Pinch of white or black pepper
1 teaspoon chopped fresh
    tarragon, parsley or
    chives, or a combination

•   Melt the butter in a non-stick frying pan over a medium heat. Pour in the eggs. Cook for 1 minute without stirring.

    With a wooden spoon or heat-resistant rubber spatula, gently turn the eggs from bottom to top, scraping around all the edges of the pan. The eggs should not brown. When the eggs form soft, creamy small curds, add herbs, turn on to warm plates and serve them immediately.

Serves 2

* for an explanation of Net Carbs see page 18.

• Ham and Swiss Cheese Frittata •

Feel free to substitute chopped smoked turkey for the ham and vary the cheese according to your taste.

NET CARBS PER SERVING: 3 grams

CARBOHYDRATES PER SERVING: 3 grams

1 tablespoon butter
½ small onion, chopped
½ pepper, chopped
1 cup chopped cooked ham
3 tablespoons chopped Italian
    (flat leaf) parsley,
    divided

9 eggs, beaten
½ cup mixed cream and milk
½ teaspoon salt
½ teaspoon Italian mixed
    herbs
1 cup grated Swiss cheese

• Heat the grill. Melt the butter in a large non-stick frying pan over a medium-high heat. Add the onion, pepper, ham, and half of the chopped parsley. Cook for 5 minutes, until the onion is softened.

Combine the eggs, cream and milk, salt, Italian mixed herbs and half the cheese. Add the egg mixture to the pan. Cook, stirring constantly until the eggs form soft, creamy small curds. This should take about five minutes. Remove from the heat and sprinkle the remaining cheese over the top of the eggs.

Place the frying pan under the grill. Cook until the cheese is bubbly and golden, which will take about 3 minutes. Cool slightly. To remove the frittata whole, tip the frying pan to one side and use a spatula to loosen the edges. Slide on to a serving platter; top with remaining parsley. Cut into wedges.

Serves 6

• Creamy Scrambled Eggs with Dill •
and Smoked Salmon

The addition of fresh dill and smoked salmon turns scrambled eggs into a special treat. Serve with buttered, toasted Atkins bread slices.

NET CARBS PER SERVING: 5 grams

CARBOHYDRATES PER SERVING: 5 grams

8 eggs
3 tablespoons cream
1 tablespoon chopped fresh dill
½ teaspoon salt
4 tablespoons butter

4 spring onions (white and 5-cm green), thinly sliced
175 g thinly sliced smoked salmon, cut into strips

• In a large bowl, beat the eggs, cream, dill, and salt. Melt the butter in a large frying pan over a medium heat. Add the spring onions. Cook for 8 minutes, until they're softened.

Pour in the egg mixture. Cook for 3 to 4 minutes, stirring occasionally, until they're almost set. Mix in the salmon and cook for 1 minute more or until eggs reach desired doneness. Transfer to warmed plates.

Serves 4

• Baked Eggs in Bacon Rings •

These baked eggs are the perfect main course for a lazy brunch with the Sunday paper.

NET CARBS PER SERVING: *3 grams*	
CARBOHYDRATES PER SERVING: *3.6 grams*	

6 rashers bacon	4 eggs
melted butter for brushing the tins	salt and pepper to taste
4 slices tomato, each about 1-cm thick	soured cream as an accompaniment (optional)

- **Preheat the oven to 160°C/325°F, gas mark 3.**

Cook the bacon in a frying pan over a medium heat until it begins to shrivel, about 3 minutes. Remove from the heat. Brush 4 cups in a muffin tin or four 140-g ramekins with the melted butter. Place a tomato slice in the bottom of each. Circle the inside of each with 1½ rashers of bacon. Break an egg into each muffin cup and season with salt and pepper. (Fill any unused cups with water to protect them from burning.) Bake in the oven for 20 minutes.

To serve, loosen the edges with a spatula and transfer the eggs to plates. Top each egg with a dollop of soured cream if desired.

Serves 2

• Eggs Benedict with Spinach •

Eggs Benedict and Eggs Florentine combine in this savoury dish.
Serve as a lunch or brunch main course.

> **NET CARBS PER SERVING:** *2.7 grams*
>
> **CARBOHYDRATES PER SERVING:** *7 grams*

4 slices uncooked smoked ham
450 g thawed and cooked
    frozen or fresh spinach
4 poached eggs
50 ml Quick & Easy
    Hollandaise Sauce (page
    180)

2 teaspoons chopped fresh
    flat-leaf parsley or dill
    for garnish (optional)

• Heat a frying pan over a medium heat until hot but not smoking. Add the ham and cook for about 2 minutes on each side, until lightly browned. Divide the spinach between 2 plates. Top each serving with 2 pieces of bacon and 2 poached eggs. Spoon the Hollandaise over the eggs and sprinkle with parsley if desired. Serve immediately.

Serves 2

Variation: For a different taste, substitute 2 thin slices of smoked salmon for the ham.

• Carrot and Nut Muffins •

These tender muffins can be made ahead and frozen, though nothing beats a freshly baked batch. What a great aroma to wake up to!

NET CARBS PER SERVING: *6 grams*

CARBOHYDRATES PER SERVING: *9 grams*

1 scant cup soy flour
1 scant cup finely ground
   almonds
1½ cups granular sugar
   substitute (do not use
   Equal or aspartame; they
   lose their sweetness when
   heated)
2 teaspoons cinnamon

1 teaspoon salt
1 teaspoon baking soda
½ teaspoon baking powder
1 cup vegetable oil
4 eggs
1 medium carrot, coarsely
   grated
2 teaspoons vanilla extract

• Heat your oven to 350°F. Grease two 6-cup muffin tins and set them aside. In a large bowl whisk together the bake mix, ground almonds, sugar substitute, cinnamon, salt, baking soda, and baking powder.

In a medium bowl, combine the vegetable oil, eggs, carrot, and vanilla extract. Pour the carrot mixture into the bake mix mixture. Stir well. Divide the batter in to the muffin tins.

Bake for 20 to 25 minutes until they're golden brown, and a cake tester inserted in to the centres of the muffins comes out clean. Cool on wire rack.

Serves 12

• Mini Chocolate Chip Muffins •

A quarter-cup of ground pecans, or your favourite nut, can be added to these muffins to make them even yummier.

> NET CARBS PER SERVING: 2.5 grams
>
> CARBOHYDRATES PER SERVING: 5 grams

1 cup soy flour
¼ cup granular sugar substitute
   (do not use Equal or
   aspartame; they lose their
   sweetness when heated)
¼ teaspoon salt
½ cup sour cream

2 tablespoons butter, melted
   and cooled
2 tablespoons heavy cream
2 tablespoons water
1 teaspoon vanilla extract
½ cup sugar-free chocolate
   chips

• Heat your oven to 350°F. Grease two 12-compartment mini muffin pans. In a bowl, whisk the bake mix, sugar substitute and salt to combine. In another bowl, whisk the sour cream, butter, heavy cream, water and vanilla to combine.

Add the sour cream mixture to the bake mix mixture. Stir until well combined. Fold in the chocolate chips. Divide the batter in to the pan compartments, using about 1 rounded table-spoon per muffin.

Bake for 15 minutes, or until the muffins are lightly browned on top and a toothpick inserted in the centre of a muffin comes out clean. Cool the muffins in their pans for 10 minutes, then turn them out on to wire racks to cool completely.

Makes 24

• Blueberry Breakfast Scones •

Nothing says 'summer' like these fresh berry scones. You may prepare the dough ahead of time, but for best results, bake just before serving.

> NET CARBS PER SERVING: 10.5 grams
>
> CARBOHYDRATES PER SERVING: 16 grams

1 cup soy flour
½ cup pecan halves
3 tablespoons plus 2 teaspoons granular sugar substitute (do not use Equal or aspartame; they lose their sweetness when heated)
1 teaspoon salt

6 tablespoons cold butter, cut into small pieces
1⅔ cups heavy cream
¼ cup sour cream
1 egg
3 cups mixed fresh berries, such as strawberries, blueberries, raspberries

• In a food processor, pulse the soy flour, pecans, 3 tablespoons of the sugar substitute and salt until the nuts are finely ground. (If you don't have a food processor, grind the nuts in a nut or coffee grinder.) Add the butter and pulse until the butter pieces are the size of peas.

In a liquid measuring cup or bowl, whisk ⅔ cup of the heavy cream, sour cream and egg. Pour evenly over the dry mixture and pulse until just combined. Transfer the dough to a baking sheet.

Separate the dough into 12 equal-sized pieces (you'll need about 3½ tablespoons of dough for each piece). Pat each piece into a disk measuring 7-cm across. Space the disks evenly on your baking sheet and chill in a refrigerator for 30 minutes. (Dough may be kept for 1 day at this point.)

Heat your oven to 375°F. Bake the shortcakes for about 17 minutes, until the bottoms are golden brown. Cool on a baking sheet set on a wire rack.

With an electric mixer on medium speed, beat the remaining cup of heavy cream with the remaining 2 teaspoons of sugar substitute until soft peaks form.

To assemble: Dollop ¼ cup of whipped cream on 6 shortcakes, top with ½ cup of berries and cover with the remaining shortcakes.

Serves 6

Hors d'oeuvre, Appetizers and Snacks

•

Guacamole

Marinated Goat's Cheese with Oregano

Courgette Rolls with Goat's Cheese

Artichoke Hearts Wrapped in Bacon

Caponata

Baked Goat's Cheese and Ricotta Custards

Devilled Eggs

Baked Brie with Sun Dried Tomatoes and Pine Nuts

Smoked Salmon Rolls

Chicken Liver Pâté with Cloves

Salmon-Stuffed Courgettes

• Guacamole •

Guacamole is not just a dip any more. This spicy Mexican specialty makes a tasty topping for an omelette or a colourful bed for grilled chicken.

> NET CARBS PER SERVING: *9.8 grams*
>
> CARBOHYDRATES PER SERVING: *10.3 grams*

1 Haas avocado, cut into
    1-cm cubes
50 g finely chopped onion
75 g chopped tomato
1 teaspoon chopped jalapeño
    chilli pepper (optional)

3 tablespoons chopped fresh
    coriander
1 tablespoon fresh lime juice
1 tablespoon olive oil
salt and pepper to taste

• Combine the avocado, onion, tomato, jalapeño pepper, if using, coriander, lime juice, oil, salt and pepper in a bowl, and mix gently. Serve immediately or store, covered, in the refrigerator for up to 2 days.

Serves 2

• Marinated Goat's Cheese • with Fresh Oregano

Goat's cheese is a firm favourite, and partnered with fresh oregano, it makes a great Mediterranean starter.

> NET CARBS PER SERVING: *1 gram*
>
> CARBOHYDRATES PER SERVING: *1 grams*

2 tablespoons extra virgin olive oil

1 tablespoon fresh oregano leaves*

½ teaspoon freshly ground pepper

1 log (200 g) goat's cheese

• Place the oil, oregano and pepper in a narrow serving dish. Roll the cheese in a mixture to coat and marinate for one hour at room temperature or refrigerate for up to 5 days.

Serves 6

* if you can't find fresh oregano leaves, substitute 1 teaspoon dried oregano.

• Courgette Rolls with Goat's Cheese •

Courgette rolls make a lovely appetizer or hors d'oeuvre. You can substitute other soft cheeses, such as cream cheese or ricotta, for the goat's cheese.

> NET CARBS PER SERVING: 5.6 grams
>
> CARBOHYDRATES PER SERVING: 6.5 grams

2 large courgettes, cut
    lengthways into six
    1-cm-thick slices
2 tablespoons olive oil
45 g creamy goat's cheese,
    softened

2 tablespoons chopped tomato
2 tablespoons chopped fresh
    flat-leaf parsley
salt and pepper to taste

• Preheat the grill.

Brush the courgette slices with the oil and grill for 2 to 3 minutes on each side, or until lightly browned. Let the courgettes cool slightly and spread each slice with 1½ teaspoons of goat's cheese. Top with 1 teaspoon of chopped tomato and 1 teaspoon of parsley, and season with salt and pepper. Roll up the courgette slices, swiss-roll style, and secure with cocktail sticks. Serve immediately.

Serves 2

• Artichoke Hearts Wrapped • in Bacon

These easy-to-prepare artichoke hearts are fabulous hors d'oeuvre or snacks.

> **NET CARBS PER PIECE:** *1.3 grams*
>
> **CARBOHYDRATES PER PIECE:** *1.5 grams*

115 g thin rashers bacon
one 400-g can artichoke
       hearts, drained and cut
       in half

- Preheat the grill.

Cut the bacon rashers in half, place on a baking sheet, and grill for 3 minutes. Let the bacon cool.

When the bacon is cool enough to handle, wrap each artichoke half in a piece of bacon, grilled side facing inward, and secure with a cocktail stick. Grill 4 to 5 minutes, or until the bacon is brown and crisp. Serve immediately.

Serves 2

• Caponata •

This Italian aubergine appetizer is delicious tucked into small endive leaves. It may be refrigerated for up to 3 days.

NET CARBS PER SERVING: 4 grams

CARBOHYDRATES PER SERVING: 5.5 grams

¼ cup extra virgin olive oil
1 medium aubergine or 2
    Italian aubergines (about
    350 g), peeled and cut
    into 0.5-cm cubes
½ red pepper
½ small onion, finely chopped
1 large clove garlic, crushed
¼ cup water
1 packet brown sugar
    substitute (do not use
    Equal or aspartame; they

lose their sweetness when
    heated)
2 tablespoons fresh lemon
    juice
1 teaspoon salt
2 tablespoons drained capers
2 tablespoons chopped fresh
    parsley leaves

• In a large saucepan, heat the olive oil over a medium heat and add the aubergine, pepper, onion, garlic and water and bring to a boil. Cover and simmer until the aubergine is tender and most of the liquid has evaporated, about 15 minutes. Stir occasionally.

Mix in the brown sugar substitute, lemon juice, salt, capers and parsley. Cool to room temperature.

Serves 6

• Baked Goat's Cheese and •
Ricotta Custards

Baked in individual ramekins, these savoury custards are wrapped in spinach leaves. Serve them on mixed greens as a first course or luncheon main course.

> NET CARBS PER SERVING: 3.5 grams
>
> CARBOHYDRATES PER SERVING: 4.5 grams

butter for greasing the
   ramekins
115 g whole-milk ricotta
   cheese
85 g fresh goat's cheese
1½ tablespoons grated
   Parmesan cheese
1½ tablespoons coarsely
   chopped walnuts

1 tablespoon chopped fresh
   basil leaves
1 egg, lightly beaten
salt and pepper to taste
6 large spinach leaves,
   stemmed and washed

• Preheat the oven to 180°/350°F, gas mark 4.
Generously butter two 150-ml ramekins.

Combine the ricotta, goat's cheese, Parmesan, walnuts, basil, egg, salt and pepper in a bowl and mix well. Line each ramekin with 3 spinach leaves. Add the cheese mixture to the ramekins, filling them three-quarters full, and bake for 30 minutes. Let the ramekins cool for 5 minutes.

To serve, place a small serving plate on top of each ramekin and turn the ramekins upside down, cutting away any spinach that overlaps the rims. Tap the bottom of the ramekins, then remove them, releasing the custards. The ramekins should slide off easily. Serve immediately.

Serves 2

• Devilled Eggs •

These tangy stuffed eggs make a surefire appetizer or snack. You may want to double or triple the recipe when entertaining — they'll disappear very quickly.

NET CARBS PER SERVING: *2 grams*

CARBOHYDRATES PER SERVING: *2 grams*

3 hard-boiled eggs
2 teaspoons finely chopped
    capers
1 tablespoon finely chopped
    celery
1 tablespoon finely chopped
    spring onion (white part
    only)
25 g boiled ham, finely

chopped
1 tablespoon mayonnaise
½ teaspoon Dijon mustard
salt and pepper to taste
paprika for garnish (optional)
chopped fresh flat-leaf parsley
    or chopped fresh dill for
    garnish (optional)

• Cut the eggs in half, remove the yolks, and place them in a bowl. Reserve the whites. Add the capers, celery, spring onions, ham, mayonnaise, mustard, salt and pepper to the egg yolks and mix well.

Divide the yolk mixture evenly among the reserved whites, mounding it slightly. Garnish the devilled eggs with paprika and parsley if desired. Serve immediately or store, covered, in the refrigerator for up to 1 day.

Serves 2

• Baked Brie with •
Sun-Dried Tomatoes and Pine Nuts

Brie with crackers is good; slightly melted Brie accented with sun-dried tomatoes and the soft crunch of pine nuts is even better. This tried-and-true appetizer never goes out of style. Serve with low-carb crackers.

> NET CARBS PER SERVING: *0.5 grams*
>
> CARBOHYDRATES PER SERVING: *0.5 grams*

1 round (225 g) Brie
1 tablespoon finely chopped
    sun-dried tomatoes in oil

1 tablespoon chopped fresh
    parsley
1 tablespoon pine nuts

• Heat the oven to 450°F. With a sharp knife, trim the white rind off the top of the cheese and place cheese in a pie plate. Mix the sun-dried tomatoes and parsley. Spread evenly over surface of cheese and sprinkle with pine nuts.

Bake for 10 minutes until heated through.

Serves 6

• Smoked Salmon Rolls •

These elegant hors d'oeuvre are delicate and flavoursome. Serve
them with a drizzling of lemon juice if desired.

NET CARBS PER SERVING: *0.8 grams*

CARBOHYDRATES PER SERVING: *0.9 grams*

50 g thinly sliced smoked
    salmon
about 2 tablespoons
    Horseradish Cream
    (page 177)

about 1 tablespoon capers
1 teaspoon chopped fresh dill

• Cut the salmon into 2.5-cm strips. Put a small dollop of horseradish cream on one end of the salmon strip and top with a caper
and a sprinkling of dill. Roll up the salmon strips, swiss-roll style,
and secure with cocktail sticks. Serve immediately.

Serves 2

• Chicken Liver Pâté with Cloves •

Pâté is an elegant hors d'oeuvre as well as an easy, delicious snack. For a sumptuous twist on the traditional devilled egg, try using this chicken liver pâté as a filling for hard-boiled egg whites.

> NET CARBS: 4.4 grams per 150g
>
> CARBOHYDRATES: 4.4 grams per 150g

115 g chicken livers
25 g butter, softened
1/4 teaspoon mustard powder
1/8 teaspoon ground cloves
1 tablespoon grated onion

pinch of cayenne pepper
salt and black pepper to taste
2 teaspoons dry sherry
  (optional)

• Place the chicken livers in a saucepan. Add enough water to just cover them, bring to a boil, and lower the heat. Simmer the livers, covered, for 15 to 20 minutes, or until tender. Drain the livers and transfer to a food processor.

Add the butter, mustard powder, cloves, onion, cayenne, salt, black pepper and sherry, if using. Purée, scraping down the side, for 1 minute, or until smooth. Transfer the pâté to a bowl and chill for 10 minutes. Serve immediately or store, covered, in the refrigerator for up to 3 days.

Makes about 150 g

• Salmon-Stuffed Courgettes •

This tasty dish is wonderful for parties as you can prepare up to six hours ahead. Smoked whitefish may be substituted for salmon.

> NET CARBS PER SERVING: *1 gram*
>
> CARBOHYDRATES PER SERVING: *1.5 grams*

2 medium or 3 small
   courgettes, scrubbed
1 tin (175 g) salmon, drained
   and flaked
2 tablespoons mayonnaise

1 teaspoon Dijon mustard
1 teaspoon chopped dill
a dash of Worcestershire sauce
1 tablespoon finely chopped
   red pepper

• With a vegetable peeler, peel stripes down the length of the courgette (to create a pattern of dark and light green). Cut the courgette into 2-cm slices; remove seeds and hollow slightly with a spoon. Arrange in rows on a serving plate.

Mix the salmon, mayonnaise, mustard, dill and Worcestershire sauce and fill the courgette hollows with the salmon mixture. Sprinkle red pepper on top of the salmon.

Serves 8

Soups

•

Cucumber Dill Soup

Manhattan Clam Chowder

Roasted Pepper Soup

French Onion Soup Gratinée

Asparagus and Leek Soup

Golden Cauliflower-Curry Soup

Roasted Vegetable Soup

Blue Cheese and Bacon Soup

• Cucumber Dill Soup •

During the warm-weather months we keep a container of this refreshing soup in the refrigerator for a quick afternoon snack.

> NET CARBS: 7.7 grams per 500ml
>
> CARBOHYDRATES: 11.2 grams per 500ml

1 tablespoon olive oil
50 g chopped onion
1 large cucumber, peeled,
    seeded, and cut into
    1-cm slices
250 ml chicken stock

1 tablespoon balsamic vinegar
7 tablespoons chopped fresh
    dill
salt and pepper to taste
soured cream as an accom-
    paniment (optional)

• Heat the oil in a large saucepan over a medium-high heat until hot but not smoking. Add the onion and sauté, stirring, for 2 minutes. Add the cucumber and stock, and bring to a boil. Lower the heat, cover, and simmer for 10 minutes. Stir in the vinegar, dill, salt and pepper.

Transfer the mixture to a food processor and purée for 1 minute, or until smooth. Serve chilled with the soured cream if desired.

Makes about 500 ml

• Manhattan Clam Chowder •

This garlicky tomato seafood soup can be put together quickly with mostly pantry ingredients. For a different flavour, try substituting the clams with prawns.

> NET CARBS PER SERVING: 6 grams
>
> CARBOHYDRATES PER SERVING: 7.5 grams

4 slices bacon, chopped
½ medium onion, chopped
2 stalks celery, chopped
2 cloves garlic, chopped
½ teaspoon dried thyme
1 tin (400 g) chopped
    tomatoes
1 medium courgette, cut into
    1-cm cubes

1 tin (400 g) vegetable broth
1 bottle (225 g) clam juice
2 tins (185 g each) chopped
    clams, undrained
salt and pepper
2 tablespoons chopped fresh
    parsley

- Cook the bacon in a large saucepan over medium heat until the fat is released. Add the onion, celery, garlic and thyme. Cook for 8 minutes, stirring occasionally, until vegetables are softened.

Stir in the tomatoes, courgette, broth and clam juice and cook for 10 minutes, until the courgette is tender. Add the clams with their juice and cook for 1 minute, to heat through. Season to taste with salt and pepper and sprinkle with parsley before serving.

Serves 6

· Roasted Pepper Soup ·

Tangy Parmesan and sweet roasted peppers make this soup flavoursome and satisfying.

> NET CARBS: *14.2 grams per 575 ml*
>
> CARBOHYDRATES: *19.2 grams per 575 ml*

2 tablespoons olive oil
1 celery stick, trimmed and
    chopped
50 g chopped onion
1 clove garlic, finely chopped
2 roasted yellow or red
    peppers (see procedure on
    page 157), peeled,
    seeded and chopped

350 ml chicken stock
75 ml double cream
salt and black pepper to taste
25 g grated Parmesan cheese

• Heat the oil in a frying pan over a moderate heat until hot but not smoking. Add the celery, onion and garlic, and cook, stirring occasionally, for about 5 minutes, until the celery is soft. Add the peppers and stock. Bring to the boil, then lower the heat and simmer for 3 minutes.

Transfer the mixture to a food processor. Add the cream, salt and pepper, and process for about 45 seconds, until smooth. Ladle the soup into 2 serving bowls and sprinkle with Parmesan. Serve immediately.

Makes about 575 ml

• French Onion Soup Gratinée •

This comforting soup is one of our all-time favourites. Serve it with Mixed Green Salad with Warm Bacon Dressing (page 70) for a cosy, satisfying supper.

> NET CARBS PER SERVING: 7.7 grams
>
> CARBOHYDRATES PER SERVING: 8.5 grams

1 tablespoon olive oil
1 medium onion, thinly sliced
one 400 ml can chicken stock
1 tablespoon Worcestershire
    sauce
½ cube of beef bouillon

2 tablespoons dry sherry
25 g grated Parmesan cheese
salt and pepper to taste
50 g Gruyère, grated
nutmeg to taste

• Preheat the grill.

Heat the oil in a large saucepan over a medium-low heat until hot but not smoking. Add the onion and cook, stirring occasionally, for 10 minutes, or until golden. Raise the heat to medium-high and add the chicken stock, Worcestershire sauce, bouillon and sherry. Bring to a boil, then lower the heat and simmer for 3 minutes. Add the Parmesan, salt and pepper, and simmer for another 3 minutes.

Transfer the soup to 2 large flameproof bowls and top each with half of the Gruyère. Grill for 3 to 4 minutes, until the cheese is melted and golden brown. Sprinkle the soup with nutmeg and serve immediately.

Serves 2

· Asparagus and Leek Soup ·

Here's a simple soup in which the taste of the vegetables really comes through. Recipes often call for a soup such as this to be strained, but I prefer the earthy texture of the more rustic version.

NET CARBS: *12.6 grams per 750 ml*

CARBOHYDRATES: *16.6 grams per 750ml*

25 g butter
1 leek (white part only),
   halved lengthways,
   washed well, and
   chopped

350 g asparagus, cut into
   1-cm pieces
500 ml chicken stock
75 ml double cream
salt and pepper to taste

• Heat the butter in a large saucepan over a medium-high heat until the foam subsides. Add the leek and sauté, stirring, for 2 minutes. Add the asparagus and sauté, stirring, for 1 minute. Add the stock to the pan and bring to the boil. Lower the heat, cover, and simmer for 8 to 10 minutes, or until the asparagus is tender.

Transfer the mixture to a food processor. Add the cream, salt and pepper, and purée for 1 minute, or until smooth. Serve immediately.

Makes about 750 ml

· Golden Cauliflower-Curry Soup ·

Spice-savvy chefs in India have long partnered cauliflower with curry and ginger. Once you try this soup, you'll see why.

> NET CARBS PER SERVING: 7.5 *grams*
>
> CARBOHYDRATES PER SERVING: 12 *grams*

1 tablespoon olive oil
1 medium onion, finely
    chopped
1 tablespoon curry powder
2 cloves garlic, finely chopped
1 teaspoon grated fresh ginger
1 medium-size head
    cauliflower, separated
    into small florets

1 tin (400 g) reduced-sodium
    chicken broth, plus 2
    cups water
1 cup heavy cream (optional)
salt and pepper
¼ cup chopped fresh chives

• Heat the oil in a large saucepan over a medium heat. Add the onion and cook for 3 minutes, until softened. Stir in curry powder, garlic and ginger; cook whilst stirring for 1 minute.

Add the cauliflower, chicken broth and water and bring to a boil over a high heat. Reduce heat to low, cover and cook for 20 minutes, or until the cauliflower is very tender. Stir in cream.

Purée the soup in batches in a blender or food processor until smooth. Return the soup to the saucepan and season to taste with salt and pepper. Heat through before serving; garnish with chives.

Serves 6

• Roasted Vegetable Soup •

A medley of flavoursome vegetables makes a pleasing first course for a holiday dinner. This soup can be made up to two days ahead. If it thickens too much, simply add a little extra chicken broth.

> **NET CARBS PER SERVING:** *9 grams*
>
> **CARBOHYDRATES PER SERVING:** *12.5 grams*

4 plum tomatoes, halved
2 small aubergines (about
    450 g each), quartered
    lengthwise
6 green onions, white and
    2.5-cm green
4 garlic cloves
3 tablespoons olive oil
1½ tablespoons fresh

marjoram or 1¼
    teaspoons dried
2 tins (400 g each) reduced
    sodium chicken broth
1 cup heavy cream (optional)
¾ teaspoon salt
½ teaspoon pepper

• Heat the oven to 400°F. Place the tomatoes, aubergines, green onions and garlic in a shallow roasting pan. Toss with oil and marjoram. Roast, turning occasionally, for 40 minutes until vegetables are tender and starting to brown.

When the aubergines are cool enough to handle, scoop out the pulp into a large saucepan; add remaining vegetables. Stir in broth. Bring to the boil over a high heat. Reduce the heat to low and simmer for 35 minutes until the vegetables are very soft. Cool.

Purée the soup in blender in batches. Return soup to saucepan and stir in cream, salt and pepper. Heat through.

Serves 8

· Blue Cheese and Bacon Soup ·

Cheese soups are especially savoury, and this one is made even more delicious with the addition of the smoky flavour of bacon. If you are not a fan of blue cheese, you can substitute an equal amount of grated Cheddar.

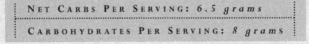

NET CARBS PER SERVING: 6.5 grams

CARBOHYDRATES PER SERVING: 8 grams

25 g butter
2 leeks (white part only),
  halved lengthways,
  washed well, and
  chopped
50 g sliced mushrooms

½ small cauliflower, broken
  into florets
350 ml chicken stock
75 g blue cheese, crumbled
6 rashers bacon, cooked and
  crumbled

• Heat the butter in a large saucepan over a medium heat until the foam subsides. Add the leeks, mushrooms and cauliflower. Cover and cook, stirring occasionally, for 5 minutes. Add the stock and bring to the boil. Lower the heat, cover, and simmer for 10 minutes.

Transfer the mixture to a food processor. Add the blue cheese and purée for 1 minute, or until smooth. Serve immediately with the crumbled bacon on top.

Serves 6

Salads

•

Orange Daikon Salad

Fennel Salad with Parmesan

Endive Salad with Walnuts and Roquefort

Walnut Coleslaw

Celeriac Salad

Red Cabbage Salad with Feta and Dill

Greek Salad

Mixed Green Salad with Warm Bacon Dressing

Warm Spinach Salad with Bacon and Pine Nuts

Open Sesame Broccoli Salad

Salad Niçoise

Tri-Colour Salad

Shrimp Cocktail with Two Sauces

Fresh Greens with Classic Vinaigrette

• Orange Daikon Salad •

Crisp, light daikon radish is a perfect ingredient for an easy, refreshing salad. If you can't find daikon, you can substitute jicama for an equally pleasing texture.

> NET CARBS PER SERVING: *3 grams*
>
> CARBOHYDRATES PER SERVING: *4.7 grams*

225 g peeled and sliced
    daikon radish or jicama
    (available at specialty
    produce markets and
    some supermarkets)

2 tablespoons sunflower oil
1 tablespoon red wine vinegar
1 teaspoon grated orange zest
salt to taste

• Place the daikon in a bowl. In another bowl, whisk together the oil, vinegar, orange zest and salt until the dressing is well blended. Pour the dressing over the daikon, toss the salad well, and serve immediately.

Serves 2

• Fennel Salad with Parmesan •

This is one of my favourite summer salads. The flavours are clean and fresh, and the Parmesan gives it just the right saltiness. For an elegant presentation, use a vegetable peeler to shave the Parmesan into paper-thin slices.

NET CARBS PER SERVING: 3.8 grams
CARBOHYDRATES PER SERVING: 4.3 grams

1 tablespoon white wine
   vinegar
3 tablespoons olive oil
salt and pepper to taste
1 tablespoon chopped fresh
   dill
1 tablespoon chopped fresh
   flat-leaf parsley

4 small fennel bulbs, halved
   lengthways, cored, and
   very thinly sliced
8 shavings of Parmesan cheese
   or 2 tablespoons grated
   Parmesan cheese

• Place the vinegar, oil, salt, pepper, dill and parsley in a small bowl. Whisk until the dressing is smooth. Place the fennel in a large bowl. Add the dressing and toss gently. Divide the salad between 2 serving plates and serve with the Parmesan.

Serves 2

· Endive Salad with Walnuts · and Roquefort

The pretty presentation of this salad makes it ideal for a special-occasion meal. You can double or triple the recipe as needed.

> NET CARBS PER SERVING: 3.8 grams
>
> CARBOHYDRATES PER SERVING: 5.4 grams

2 tablespoons olive oil
1 teaspoon fresh lemon juice
1 teaspoon fresh orange juice
1 teaspoon grated orange zest
30 g crumbled Roquefort or
    other blue cheese
salt and pepper to taste

1 plump head of endive, leaves
    separated, washed well,
    and spun dry
30 g chopped walnuts, lightly
    toasted (see Hint on
    page 172)

• Whisk together the oil, lemon juice, orange juice, orange zest, Roquefort, salt and pepper in a small bowl. (If the cheese clumps, mash it with a fork.) Arrange the endive leaves on a serving plate like the spokes of a wheel. Pour the Roquefort dressing over the endive and sprinkle with the walnuts. Serve immediately.

Serves 2

· Walnut Coleslaw ·

Crunchy and fresh, this salad of sprouts and walnuts is a delicious twist on the more traditional recipe.

> NET CARBS PER SERVING: *1.6 grams*
>
> CARBOHYDRATES PER SERVING: *3.8 grams*

50 g chopped cabbage	1 tablespoon Dijon mustard
50 g alfalfa sprouts	1 teaspoon balsamic vinegar
25 g chopped walnuts	salt and pepper to taste
50 ml mayonnaise	

- **Combine the cabbage, sprouts, walnuts, mayonnaise, mustard, vinegar, salt and pepper in a large bowl. Mix well. Serve immediately.**

Serves 2

• Celeriac Salad •

Celeriac has a clean flavour and crunchy texture. It's a seasonal vegetable, not available year-round, but an equal amount of chopped celery can be substituted. Serve this salad with Spiced Steak (page 130).

> **NET CARBS PER SERVING:** *0.2 grams*
>
> **CARBOHYDRATES PER SERVING:** *4.4 grams*

2 tablespoons mayonnaise
1 teaspoon Dijon mustard
2 teaspoons balsamic vinegar
salt and pepper to taste

140 g peeled and coarsely
    chopped celeriac
1 tablespoon chopped fresh
    coriander or parsley

• **Combine the mayonnaise, mustard, vinegar, salt, pepper and celeriac in a bowl and mix well. Sprinkle with the coriander and serve immediately.**

Serves 2

• Red Cabbage Salad with • Feta and Dill

A friend created this colourful salad for a potluck dinner, and ever since it has been her most requested dish for informal get-togethers and picnics.

> **NET CARBS PER SERVING: 5.5 grams**
>
> **CARBOHYDRATES PER SERVING: 8.1 grams**

50 ml olive oil
juice of ½ lemon
1 clove garlic, finely chopped
salt and pepper to taste
170 g chopped red cabbage

45 g pine nuts, lightly toasted
  (see Hint on page 172)
115 g crumbled feta cheese
6 tablespoons chopped fresh
  dill

• Whisk together the oil, lemon juice, garlic, salt and pepper in a large serving bowl. Add the cabbage, pine nuts, feta and dill, and toss well. Serve immediately.

Serves 2

• Greek Salad •

This snappy salad makes a delicious lunch or first course.

NET CARBS PER SERVING: *5.4 grams*

CARBOHYDRATES PER SERVING: *7.8 grams*

1 medium tomato, cut into
    5-cm pieces
1 cucumber, peeled, seeded and
    sliced
25 g thinly sliced red onion
75 g crumbled feta cheese

2 Kalamata olives, cut into
    slivers (optional)
3 tablespoons olive oil
1 tablespoon red wine vinegar
salt and pepper to taste

• Combine the tomato, cucumber, onion, feta and olives, if using, in a large serving bowl. Whisk together the oil, vinegar, salt and pepper in a small bowl. Pour the dressing over the salad and toss well. Serve immediately.

Serves 2

• Mixed Green Salad with •
Warm Bacon Dressing

Smoky bacon and sweet sautéed leek combine in a flavour-packed salad dressing that blends beautifully with assorted greens.

> NET CARBS PER SERVING: *4.3 grams*
>
> CARBOHYDRATES PER SERVING: *6.1 grams*

45 g bacon lardons, cut into 2.5-cm pieces
1 leek (white part only), halved lengthways, washed well, and thinly sliced crossways
3 tablespoons olive oil

1 tablespoon red wine vinegar
salt and pepper to taste
100 g assorted lettuce leaves (such as romaine and red leaf), washed and spun dry

• Sauté the bacon in a heavy frying pan over a medium-high heat, stirring, for about 2 to 3 minutes, until it turns golden brown. Add the leek and sauté, stirring, for about 4 minutes. Reduce the heat to medium-low. Add the oil, vinegar, salt and pepper, and cook for 1 minute. Place the lettuce leaves in a large bowl, pour the bacon dressing over them, and toss gently. Serve immediately.

Serves 2

· Warm Spinach Salad · with Bacon and Pine Nuts

You'll love this variation on the traditional spinach salad. The texture of the pine nuts mellows the saltiness of the bacon and the tanginess of the vinegar.

NET CARBS PER SERVING: *11 grams*	
CARBOHYDRATES PER SERVING: *18 grams*	

2 tablespoons olive oil
4 rashers streaky bacon, cut into 1-cm pieces
2 tablespoons pine nuts
2 small cloves garlic, finely chopped

450 g spinach leaves, trimmed, washed well, and spun dry
1 tablespoon balsamic vinegar
1 tablespoon grated Parmesan cheese

• Heat 1 tablespoon of oil in a heavy frying pan over a medium-high heat until hot but not smoking. Add the bacon and sauté, stirring occasionally, for 4 minutes, or until browned. Reduce the heat to medium, add the pine nuts, and cook for 1 minute, stirring occasionally. Add the garlic and cook, stirring, for 30 seconds. Add the spinach, vinegar and remaining tablespoon of oil, and cook, tossing gently, for 15 seconds, or until the spinach is warm and a bit wilted. Transfer to serving plates, sprinkle with Parmesan, and serve immediately.

Serves 2

• Open Sesame Broccoli •
Salad

An unusual combination, sesame and broccoli make an attractive salad. To turn it into a main course, add sliced cooked chicken or pork.

> NET CARBS PER SERVING: *3 grams*
>
> CARBOHYDRATES PER SERVING: *5.5 grams*

2 medium heads of broccoli,
    broken into florets
    (about 8 cups)
¼ cup sesame seeds
2 tablespoons reduced sodium
    soy sauce
2 tablespoons rice vinegar

2 tablespoons dark sesame oil
1½ packets sugar substitute
    (do not use Equal or
    aspartame; they lose
    their sweetness when
    heated)

•   In a large pot of lightly salted boiling water, cook the broccoli for 5 minutes, until crisp-tender. Rinse under cold water; drain.

In a dry frying pan over medium heat, toast sesame seeds for 5 minutes, until golden and fragrant. Transfer to small plate to cool.

Combine the soy sauce, vinegar, oil and sugar substitute and mix well in a large bowl. Add the broccoli and half the sesame seeds and toss well. Marinate at room temperature at least 30 minutes, stirring occasionally. Before serving, sprinkle broccoli with remaining sesame seeds. It will keep well in the refrigerator for up to 2 days.

Serves 8

• Salad Niçoise •

This French classic always makes for a filling summer lunch. Some versions use fresh grilled tuna, but for the most flavour and authenticity, canned tuna packed in olive oil is the best bet.

> **NET CARBS PER SERVING: 9.5 grams**
>
> **CARBOHYDRATES PER SERVING: 13.5 grams**

3 tablespoons olive oil
1½ tablespoons red wine
    vinegar
1 teaspoon Dijon mustard
2 cans (175 g each) tuna in
    olive oil, lightly drained
    and flaked
2 hard-boiled eggs
1 medium tomato, quartered
    lengthwise

160 g green beans, cooked
    until tender-crisp
¼ small red onion, thinly
    sliced
6 oil-cured black olives, cut
    into slivers
4 anchovies (optional)
salt and pepper

• **In a large bowl, whisk together the olive oil and vinegar. Arrange tuna, eggs, tomatoes, green beans, and onion on two plates. Drizzle with dressing; top with olives and anchovies. Add salt and pepper to taste.**

Serves 2

· Tri-Colour Salad ·

This pretty salad is a great side dish. To make it a main course, add sliced chicken or another form of protein.

NET CARBS PER SERVING: *1.5 grams*

CARBOHYDRATES PER SERVING: *2.5 grams*

Dressing:
3 tablespoons olive oil
1 tablespoon balsamic vinegar
   (or red wine vinegar
   mixed with ½ packet
   sugar substitute — but do
   not use Equal or
   aspartame; they lose
   their sweetness when
   heated)

½ teaspoon lemon juice
½ teaspoon salt
¼ teaspoon pepper
Salad:
1 head endive, thinly sliced on
   the diagonal
½ small head radicchio, cut
   into bite-sized pieces
½ small head Bibb lettuce, cut
   into bite-sized pieces

• In a salad bowl, whisk together the olive oil, balsamic vinegar, lemon juice, salt and pepper. Add the endive, radicchio, and lettuce. Toss to coat with dressing.

Serves 4

• Shrimp Cocktail with Two Sauces •

Red and green cocktail sauces make this appetizer both festive and tasty. One is spicy, the other milder.

> NET CARBS PER SERVING: *1.5 grams*
>
> CARBOHYDRATES PER SERVING: *1.5 grams*

24 large or jumbo shrimp
2 tablespoons red Horseradish
    sauce
1 tablespoon mayonnaise
½ red pepper, coarsely
    chopped
½ teaspoon Worcestershire
    sauce
2 tablespoons green salsa

¼ cup parsley leaves, stems
    removed
1 spring onion, coarsely
    chopped
2 teaspoons olive oil
1 tablespoon chopped chives or
    finely chopped green end
    of a spring onion

• Bring a large pot of lightly salted water to the boil. Peel the shrimp (leave tails on, if desired) and remove black veins from each shrimp with a small sharp knife; rinse shrimp.

Cook the shrimp for 3 to 5 minutes just until opaque and cooked through. Remove with a slotted spoon and refresh under cold water (shrimp may be made 1 day ahead).

In a food processor or blender, process the horseradish, mayonnaise, pepper and Worcestershire sauce until fairly smooth. Transfer to a bowl; clean bowl of food processor.

Process the salsa, parsley, onion and oil until fairly smooth. On each serving plate, place 1 tablespoon of red sauce and 1 tablespoon of green sauce side by side. Spread the sauces out toward the edge of the plate with the tip of a knife. Arrange 4 shrimp in a circular pattern over the sauce and sprinkle with chopped chives.

Serves 6

• Fresh Greens with Classic •
Vinaigrette

Simple yet tasty, this is a wonderful partner for chicken.

> NET CARBS PER SERVING: *1.5 grams*
>
> CARBOHYDRATES PER SERVING: *2 grams*

¼ cup red or white wine vinegar	⅛ teaspoon pepper (preferably freshly ground)
1 teaspoon Dijon mustard	¾ cup extra-virgin olive oil
¼ teaspoon salt	6 cups spring salad mix

• In a small bowl, whisk together the vinegar, mustard, salt and pepper. Whisk in the oil in a slow, steady stream until completely incorporated. Pour ⅓ to ½ cup of the dressing over salad mix; toss well to coat. This recipe provides enough dressing for 16 cups of salad and the leftover dressing may be refrigerated for up to five days.

Herb vinaigrette: add 3 tablespoons of finely chopped herbs, such as parsley, basil or chervil (or a combination)

Lemon vinaigrette: substitute lemon juice for the vinegar; add 1 teaspoon grated lemon rind and 1 tablespoon finely chopped shallot or green onion.

Serves 8

Main Courses

•

EGGS

SEAFOOD

POULTRY

PORK

LAMB

BEEF

Eggs

•

Mustard Scrambled Eggs

Ricotta and Leek Frittata

Smoked Salmon Frittata

Herb Kookoo (Frittata with Herbs)

Egg Salad with Capers

· Mustard Scrambled Eggs ·

Dr Atkins loves to make breakfast on weekends, and he often comes up with some very unusual and tasty combinations. This is one of his favourites. Serve with bacon or sausage on the side.

> NET CARBS PER SERVING: *1.4 grams*
>
> CARBOHYDRATES PER SERVING: *1.4 grams*

4 eggs
1 teaspoon mustard powder
½ teaspoon crumbled dried
    oregano

1 tablespoon hot water
2 tablespoons soured cream
25 g butter
salt and pepper to taste

- Combine the eggs, mustard powder, oregano, water and soured cream in a bowl and beat lightly. Heat the butter in a frying pan over a medium heat until the foam subsides. Add the egg mixture and cook, stirring, about 4 minutes, until the mixture becomes custardlike but not loose. Sprinkle with salt and pepper, and serve immediately.

Serves 2

· Ricotta and Leek Frittata ·

Leeks become marvelously sweet when they are sautéed. Here, they give an extra measure of flavour to this frittata. Serve with a mixed green salad.

> NET CARBS PER SERVING: *0.9 grams*
>
> CARBOHYDRATES PER SERVING: *2 grams*

15 g butter
1 leek (white part only),
    halved lengthways,
    washed well, and cut
    into 1-cm pieces

1½ tablespoons whole-milk
    ricotta cheese
salt and pepper to taste
4 eggs, lightly beaten

- Preheat the grill.
    Heat half of the butter in a 25-cm frying pan (preferably non-stick) over a medium-high heat until the foam subsides. Add the leek and sauté, stirring, for 3 minutes. Remove from the heat and cool.
    Add the sautéed leek, ricotta, salt and pepper to the beaten eggs and mix well. Heat the remaining butter in the frying pan over a medium heat until the foam subsides. Pour in the egg mixture and cook, stirring, about 1 minute, until the egg starts to form curds. Cook for another minute (the egg mixture should be set on the bottom and still a bit wet on top).
    Place the frying pan under the grill for about 2 minutes, until the frittata turns golden brown. Using a spatula, carefully remove the frittata from the frying pan. Cut into wedges and serve.

Serves 2

· Smoked Salmon Frittata ·

Eggs are not just for breakfast. This elegant frittata is perfect for a late supper. For special occasions, serve it with soured cream and caviar.

> NET CARBS PER SERVING: *0.3 grams*
>
> CARBOHYDRATES PER SERVING: *0.3 grams*

4 large eggs, lightly beaten
25 g smoked salmon, chopped
1 teaspoon chopped fresh
    chives

1 tablespoon soured cream
salt and pepper to taste
15 g butter

- Preheat the grill.

Beat together the eggs, salmon, chives, soured cream, salt and pepper in a bowl. Heat the butter in a 25-cm frying pan (preferably nonstick) over a medium heat until the foam subsides. Pour in the egg mixture and cook, stirring, for about 1 minute, until the egg starts to form curds. Cook for another minute (the egg mixture should be set on the bottom and still a bit wet on top).

Place the frying pan under the grill and grill for about 2 minutes, until the frittata turns golden brown. Using a spatula, carefully remove the frittata from the frying pan. Cut into wedges and serve.

Serves 2

• Herb Kookoo •
(Frittata with Herbs)

No doubt about it, we are absolutely cuckoo for this Middle Eastern version of a frittata that we adapted from *Food of Life* by Najmieh Batmanglij. Kookoos and frittatas are usually served at room temperature, cut into wedges. When accompanied by a great salad, the dish makes a main course. For a variation, try using a slice of kookoo as the 'base' for an open-faced, knife-and-fork sandwich of ham and Gruyère or chicken salad.

> NET CARBS PER SERVING: *2.4 grams*
>
> CARBOHYDRATES PER SERVING: *7.1 grams*

75 g chopped spring onion (white part only)	8 large eggs
1 large bunch chopped fresh flat-leaf parsley	1/4 teaspoon freshly ground pepper
7 tablespoons chopped fresh dill	1/2 teaspoon bicarbonate of soda
7 tablespoons chopped fresh coriander	1 teaspoon salt
	50 ml olive or rapeseed oil

• **Combine the spring onion, parsley, dill and coriander in a food processor and blend for 5 seconds. Scrape down the side and add the eggs, pepper, bicarbonate of soda, salt and 2 tablespoons of the oil. Blend the mixture for about 30 seconds, or until smooth.**

Heat the remaining oil in a heavy frying pan over a medium heat until hot but not smoking. Add the egg mixture to the frying pan, cover, and cook it over a low heat for about 15 minutes, stirring once during the first 7 minutes or until it is set. Cut the kookoo into 4 wedges and turn the wedges 1 at a time. Cook the kookoo for another 5 minutes. Remove from the pan and let cool for 2 minutes. Serve immediately or store in the refrigerator for up to 2 days.

Serves 2

• Egg Salad with Capers •

You can't go wrong with this egg salad for a quick lunch. It is served on a bed of crisp lettuce.

NET CARBS PER SERVING: *0.8 gram*

CARBOHYDRATES PER SERVING: *1.1 grams*

4 hard-boiled eggs, peeled and
    chopped
2 tablespoons mayonnaise
1 teaspoon Dijon mustard
2 tablespoons chopped celery
1 tablespoon small capers or
    chopped large capers

½ teaspoon chopped fresh
    tarragon or ¼ teaspoon
    crumbled dried tarragon
salt and pepper to taste

• Combine the eggs, mayonnaise, mustard, celery, capers, tarragon, salt and pepper in a bowl and mix well. Serve or store, covered, in the refrigerator for up to 1 day.

Serves 2

Seafood

•

Scallops with Thyme

Thai Coconut-Ginger Shrimp

Stir-Fried Prawns with Ginger and Mushrooms

Prawn Scampi

Tarragon Prawn Salad

Crab and Avocado Salad

Sautéed Cod with Lemon-Parsley Sauce

Red Snapper with Tomato and Olives

Mackerel Fillets with Mustard-Rosemary Mayonnaise

Fish Fillets with Tomatoes and Black Olives

Mahi-Mahi with Creole Sauce

Oven-Poached Salmon with Dill and Wine

Cajun Blackened Tuna

Peppers Stuffed with Walnut Tuna Salad

Pepper-Crusted Swordfish

Squid with Basil and Lime

• Scallops with Thyme •

The rich, succulent flavour of scallops is complemented here by the tangy lemon and fresh thyme. Serve with Orange Daikon Salad (page 63).

NET CARBS PER SERVING: 8.8 grams

CARBOHYDRATES PER SERVING: 9.3 grams

2 teaspoons salt
1 teaspoon cayenne pepper
450 g scallops, rinsed and
    patted dry
45 g butter
2 cloves garlic, finely chopped

2 spring onions (white part
    only), chopped
1 tablespoon fresh thyme or
    1½ teaspoons crumbled
    dried thyme
juice of ½ lemon

• Combine the salt and cayenne in a small bowl. Sprinkle the mixture over the scallops. Heat the butter in a heavy frying pan or a wok over a medium-high heat until it is bubbling and beginning to brown. Add the garlic and spring onions, and cook, stirring, for 30 seconds. Add the scallops and thyme to the frying pan and cook, turning the scallops, for about 4 minutes, until they are lightly browned. Drizzle with the lemon juice and serve immediately.

Serves 2

• Thai Coconut-Shrimp •

The combination of the coconut and ginger make this tangy main dish a great favourite but be sure you buy unsweetened coconut milk (not the kind used for piña coladas), and add enough red pepper flakes to accent the creamy sauce.

NET CARBS PER SERVING: *4 grams*

CARBOHYDRATES PER SERVING: *5 grams*

2 tablespoons peanut oil
½ small onion, finely chopped
1 tablespoon peeled and grated fresh ginger
3 garlic cloves, finely chopped
⅛ teaspoon red pepper flakes (or more, to taste)
2 tomatoes, seeded and chopped

⅔ cup unsweetened coconut milk
900 g large shrimp, peeled and deveined
salt and pepper
3 tablespoons chopped fresh basil

• Heat the oil in a large non-stick frying pan over medium heat. Cook the onion for 3 minutes, until softened. Stir in the ginger, garlic, and red pepper flakes and cook for 1 minute more. Add the tomatoes and coconut milk. Cook for 10 minutes or until mixture thickens.

Add the shrimp to the frying pan. Cook for 3 to 4 minutes, until cooked through. Add salt and freshly ground black pepper to taste and sprinkle with basil before serving.

Serves 4

• Stir-Fried Prawns with • Ginger and Mushrooms

A quick and easy stir-fry is a perfect weekday supper. In this recipe you can substitute an equal amount of chicken breast for the prawns, cut into strips.

> **NET CARBS PER SERVING: 4.9 grams**
>
> **CARBOHYDRATES PER SERVING: 5.4 grams**

1 tablespoon rapeseed oil
2 cloves garlic, finely chopped
1 tablespoon peeled and chopped gingerroot
25 g sliced mushrooms
1 stick celery, chopped
1 tablespoon toasted sesame oil

1 tablespoon soy sauce
¼ teaspoon dried hot red chilli pepper flakes, or to taste
350 g prawns, shelled and deveined

• Heat the oil in a large, heavy frying pan or a wok over a medium-high heat until hot but not smoking. Add the garlic and gingerroot, and stir-fry for 30 seconds. Add the mushrooms, celery, sesame oil, soy sauce, chilli pepper flakes and prawns. Stir-fry until the prawns are pink and just cooked through, 3 to 4 minutes. Serve immediately.

Serves 2

• Prawn Scampi •

Lemon, wine and garlic do wonders for prawns. This dish is very easy to make and is always a hit. You can easily double the recipe to serve guests.

> NET CARBS PER SERVING: 6.2 grams
>
> CARBOHYDRATES PER SERVING: 6.6 grams

25 g butter
2 tablespoons olive oil
4 large cloves garlic, finely chopped
3 tablespoons chopped fresh flat-leaf parsley
juice of ½ lemon

100 ml dry white wine
pinch of dried hot red chilli pepper flakes
salt and black pepper to taste
450 g large prawns, shelled and deveined

• Heat the butter and oil in a heavy frying pan over a medium heat until the foam subsides. Add the garlic, parsley, lemon juice, wine, chilli pepper flakes, salt and pepper. Bring to the boil, lower the heat, and simmer for 3 minutes. Add the prawns to the frying pan and cook, stirring frequently, for 5 to 6 minutes, until the prawns are pink. Remove from the heat. Place the prawns on a serving plate and pour the sauce from the frying pan over them. Serve immediately.

Serves 2

· Tarragon Prawn Salad ·

Cool and refreshing, this tarragon-infused prawn salad is a perfect light luncheon. Serve it on a bed of crisp mixed greens.

NET CARBS PER SERVING: 3.4 grams

CARBOHYDRATES PER SERVING: 3.8 grams

100 ml mayonnaise
2 tablespoons Dijon mustard
½ teaspoon Anchovy Paste
    (page 168) or 1 oil-
    packed anchovy fillet,
    mashed
½ tablespoon small capers or
    chopped large capers
½ tablespoon chopped fresh
    flat-leaf parsley

½ tablespoon chopped fresh
    tarragon or ¾ teaspoon
    crumbled dried tarragon
salt and pepper to taste
350 g cooked medium prawns,
    shelled and deveined

• Whisk together the mayonnaise, mustard, anchovy paste, capers, parsley, tarragon, salt and pepper in a large serving bowl. Add the prawns and toss the salad well. Serve immediately.

Serves 2

· Crab and Avocado Salad ·

Sweet crabmeat and creamy avocado combine in this delectable salad with a spicy fragrance.

NET CARBS PER SERVING: 5.8 grams

CARBOHYDRATES PER SERVING: 6.1 grams

1 stick celery, chopped
225 g cooked fresh crabmeat;
    or frozen crabmeat,
    thawed, or canned
    crabmeat, drained
1 tablespoon mayonnaise
1 teaspoon cumin
½ teaspoon turmeric
1 tablespoon capers

salt and pepper to taste
juice of ½ lemon
½ medium Haas avocado,
    cubed and drizzled with
    lemon juice
1 bunch watercress, stems
    removed

• Combine the celery, crabmeat, mayonnaise, cumin, turmeric, capers, salt, pepper and lemon juice in a large bowl and mix well. Gently stir in the avocado. Divide the watercress between 2 plates, top with the crab salad, and serve immediately.

Serves 2

• Sautéed Cod with •
Lemon-Parsley Sauce

Cod has a very delicate flavour and texture, so it tends to fall apart when sautéed. Don't worry about a less-than-perfect presentation — the taste makes up for it.

> NET CARBS PER SERVING: *1.5 grams*
>
> CARBOHYDRATES PER SERVING: *3.3 grams*

15 g butter
1 tablespoon olive oil
3 cloves garlic, thinly sliced
75 g chopped onion
450 g cod fillets
juice of ½ lemon

1½ tablespoons chopped fresh
  flat-leaf parsley
1 tablespoon fresh thyme or
  1½ teaspoons crumbled
  dried thyme
salt and pepper to taste

• Heat the butter and oil in a frying pan over a medium-high heat until the foam subsides. Add the garlic and sauté, stirring, for 5 seconds. Add the onion and sauté for 1 minute. Add the cod and sauté for 5 minutes, turning once (the fish will crumble). Add the lemon juice, parsley, thyme, salt and pepper. Cover the frying pan and cook the fish for about 2 minutes, until the cod is opaque and flaky. Serve immediately.

Serves 2

· Red Snapper with Tomato · and Olives

The lusty flavours of classic Italian *puttanesca* sauce — tomatoes, capers, black olives — have a wonderful affinity for firm-fleshed red snapper. Serve with Green Beans with Garlic-Tarragon Vinaigrette (page 149).

> NET CARBS PER SERVING: *6.2 grams*
>
> CARBOHYDRATES PER SERVING: *8.2 grams*

1 tablespoon olive oil
½ small onion, chopped
1 clove garlic, finely chopped
5 Greek black olives, stoned and chopped
170 g chopped tomatoes

2 tablespoons capers
50 ml dry red wine
pinch of dried hot red chilli pepper flakes (optional)
25 g butter
675 g red snapper fillets

• Heat the oil in a large frying pan over a medium heat until hot but not smoking. Add the onion, garlic and olives. Cook, stirring occasionally, for 3 minutes, or until the onion is transparent. Add the tomatoes, capers, wine and chilli pepper flakes, if using. Bring to the boil, lower the heat, and simmer for 5 minutes.

Meanwhile, heat the butter in another large frying pan over a medium heat until the foam subsides. Cook the snapper for 2 minutes on each side, or until lightly browned. Transfer the snapper to the tomato mixture in the frying pan, cover, and cook over a medium heat for 3 minutes, or until the snapper just flakes. Serve immediately.

Serves 2

• Mackerel Fillets with •
Mustard-Rosemary Mayonnaise

Tasty, strong flavoured mackerel holds up well to assertive seasoning. This dish is for those who enjoy full flavoured fish.

> NET CARBS PER SERVING: *1 gram*
>
> CARBOHYDRATES PER SERVING: *1 gram*

4 (250 g) mackerel fillets (or bluefish fillets)

2 garlic cloves

½ teaspoon salt

½ teaspoon dried rosemary leaves

1 tablespoon Dijon mustard

¼ cup mayonnaise

• Heat the grill. On a cutting board mash garlic with salt until you have a paste. Add the rosemary leaves to the paste and chop. Transfer to a small bowl and mix in mustard and mayonnaise.

Arrange fish fillets in grill and spread evenly with rosemary-mustard mayonnaise. Grill 5 inches from heat source until cooked through, for about 8 minutes.

Serves 4

• Fish Fillets with Tomatoes •
and Black Olives

The lusty flavors of classic Italian puttanesca sauce — tomatoes, capers, black olives — have a wonderful affinity for firm-fleshed fish such as red snapper, sea bass, or even catfish.

> NET CARBS PER SERVING: *3.5 grams*
>
> CARBOHYDRATES PER SERVING: *4.5 grams*

1 tablespoon olive oil
1 small onion, chopped
10 Greek olives, pitted and
    chopped
2 plum tomatoes, chopped
2 tablespoons capers

2 garlic cloves, finely chopped
½ cup dry red wine
Pinch of dried hot red pepper
    flakes (optional)
4 tablespoons butter
2 pounds red snapper fillets

• Heat the oil in a large frying pan over a medium heat until very hot. Add the onion and olives. Cook, stirring occasionally, for 3 minutes, or until the onion is transparent. Add the tomatoes, capers, garlic, wine, and red pepper flakes, if using. Bring to the boil; reduce heat, and simmer for 5 minutes.

Meanwhile, melt the butter in another large frying pan over medium heat. Cook snapper (in batches, if necessary) for 2 minutes per side or until lightly browned. Transfer the snapper fillets to the tomato mixture in the frying pan, cover, and cook over medium heat for 3 to 4 minutes, just until fish is cooked through. Serve immediately.

Serves 4

• Mahi-Mahi with Creole Sauce •

Also called dolphin fish, mahi-mahi has a firm yet delicate texture, and stands up well to flavourful sauces. This delicious recipe is a favourite on Atkins cruises.

> NET CARBS PER SERVING: 2.5 grams
>
> CARBOHYDRATES PER SERVING: 3 grams

4 (225 g each) mahi-mahi fillets or other firm white fish
1 tablespoon fresh lemon juice
salt and pepper to taste
1 tablespoon butter
½ small onion, thinly sliced
½ small red pepper, cut in thin strips
½ small green pepper, cut in thin strips
½ cup chopped canned tomatoes, with juice
1 tablespoon chopped fresh cilantro
Hot pepper sauce, to taste
1 tablespoon olive oil

• Sprinkle the fish with lemon juice, salt and pepper and set aside. In a saucepan over medium-high heat, melt the butter. Cook the onions and peppers for 2 minutes, until barely tender.

Add the tomatoes with their juice; reduce heat to medium and simmer for 8 minutes, until sauce thickens. Stir in the cilantro and add pepper sauce to taste.

Heat the oil in a large non-stick fyring pan over high heat. Sauté the fish for 3 minutes per side, until cooked through. Transfer to a serving platter and spoon the sauce over fish.

Serves 4

• Oven-Poached Salmon with •
Dill and Wine

Fresh salmon has a very delicate flavour, and oven-poaching will keep it moist and tasty. Serve the salmon warm with lemon wedges or chilled with Cucumber-Dill Sauce (page 175), Creamy Celery Sauce (page 176) or Horseradish Cream (page 177).

NET CARBS PER SERVING: *2.2 grams*

CARBOHYDRATES PER SERVING: *2.3 grams*

450-g salmon steak (about 2.5-cm thick)
salt and pepper to taste
3 tablespoons chopped fresh dill

3 tablespoons fresh lemon or lime juice
3 tablespoons dry white wine
1 bay leaf

• **Preheat the oven to 190°C/375°F, gas mark 5. Place the salmon steak on 2 layers of aluminum foil, twice as big as the salmon. Salt and pepper the salmon. Bring up all sides of the foil and carefully add the dill, lemon juice, wine and bay leaf. Fold all sides of the foil together, creating a tent over the salmon.**

Place the salmon tent on a baking sheet and bake for 20 minutes. Remove from the oven and carefully unwrap the top of the foil (the steam will be very hot). Gently transfer the salmon to a serving plate, discarding the bay leaf. Pour any liquid in the foil over the fish. Serve immediately.

Serves 2

• Cajun Blackened Tuna •

Tuna, a naturally lean fish, is tender and juicy when cooked rare or medium-rare. In this wonderfully flavoursome dish, searing dry heat chars a spice crust on to the fish.

> **NET CARBS PER SERVING:** *1 gram*
>
> **CARBOHYDRATES PER SERVING:** *2 grams*

Spice Mixture:
1 tablespoon sweet paprika
1 teaspoon oregano
1 teaspoon garlic powder
1 teaspoon onion powder
1 teaspoon salt
½ teaspoon ground cumin
½ teaspoon freshly ground
    black pepper

¼ teaspoon cayenne pepper
    (optional)
2 tablespoons unsalted butter,
    softened
4 (250 g) tuna steaks (about
    2-cm thick each)

• Heat the oven to 400°F. Combine the paprika, oregano, garlic powder, onion powder, salt, cumin, pepper, and cayenne pepper on a plate. Rub butter over the tuna steaks. Press the steaks into the spice mixture and gently rub spices on to fish.

Heat a large heavy ovenproof frying pan (cast iron works great) over a high heat for 2 minutes or until the pan smokes. Cook the tuna steaks for 1 minute on each side. They will make some smoke – this is normal. Transfer the pan to the oven and roast the fish for 5 minutes for medium-rare doneness. If you don't have an ovenproof pan, transfer seared fish to a baking sheet to finish cooking.

Serves 4

• Peppers Stuffed with •
Walnut Tuna Salad

You'll never miss the bread with this zesty version of a quick tuna salad. For a more hearty winter lunch, add grated cheese to the top and bake for a few minutes. It makes a great tuna melt.

> **NET CARBS PER SERVING: 6.3 grams**
>
> **CARBOHYDRATES PER SERVING: 8.5 grams**

one 170-g can chunk white
    tuna, drained
25 g chopped walnuts
75 g chopped spring onion
    (white part only)
juice of ½ lemon
1 teaspoon olive oil
2 tablespoons mayonnaise
½ teaspoon Dijon mustard

¼ teaspoon white pepper
salt to taste
1 sweet pepper, cut in half and
    seeded
1 tablespoon chopped fresh
    dill (optional)
2 thin lemon slices for garnish
    (optional)

• Combine the tuna, walnuts, spring onion, lemon juice, oil, mayonnaise, mustard, white pepper and salt in a bowl and mix well. Fill each pepper half with half the tuna mixture. Sprinkle with the dill and garnish with the lemon slices if desired. Serve immediately.

Serves 2

• Pepper-Crusted Swordfish •

Meaty, rich swordfish makes a perfect foil for this spicy, aromatic crust. Serve with Cucumber-Dill Sauce (page 175).

NET CARBS PER SERVING: 3.3 grams

CARBOHYDRATES PER SERVING: 4.4 grams

350 g swordfish steak (about
    2.5-cm thick), cut into 2
    pieces
juice of ½ lime
1 tablespoon coarsely ground
    coriander seeds
2 tablespoons coarsely ground
    black peppercorns
25 g coarsely ground
    hazelnuts
salt to taste
25 g butter, softened

- **Preheat the grill.**

   Drizzle the swordfish with the lime juice and grill for 3 minutes on each side. Meanwhile, combine the coriander, peppercorns, hazelnuts and salt in a bowl and mix well. Let the swordfish cool slightly. Pat the peppercorn mixture on all sides of the fish and dot with the butter. Grill the swordfish for 4 minutes, turning once. Serve immediately.

Serves 2

• Squid with Basil and Lime •

Sweet basil blends beautifully with the mild, almost nutty flavour of squid. Squid freezes well, so if you don't have access to fresh squid, the frozen product is fine. Serve with mixed baby greens.

> NET CARBS PER SERVING: *9 grams*
>
> CARBOHYDRATES PER SERVING: *9.5 grams*

450 g cleaned squid, bodies
    cut into 1-cm rings and
    tentacles halved
7 tablespoons chopped fresh
    basil leaves
2 tablespoons olive oil

juice of 1 lime
1 clove garlic, finely chopped
¼ teaspoon dried hot red
    chilli pepper flakes
1 tablespoon peanut oil

• **Combine the squid, basil, olive oil, lime juice, garlic and chilli flakes in a bowl and mix well. Let the squid marinate, covered, in the refrigerator for at least 20 minutes and up to 1 hour.**

Heat a wok or heavy frying pan over a medium-high heat until a drop of water sizzles on the surface, about 45 seconds. Pour the peanut oil into the wok, add the squid, and cook, stirring frequently, for about 4 minutes, until the squid is opaque and tender. Serve immediately.

Serves 2

Variation: You can easily adapt this recipe to create a delightful seafood salad. Chill the Squid with Basil and Lime for 30 minutes. Add 1 stick chopped celery and half a chopped sweet pepper. Whisk together 3 tablespoons of oil and 1 tablespoon of fresh lemon juice. Drizzle the dressing over the salad, toss gently, and serve.

Poultry

•

Chicken with Lemon and Capers
Coconut Chicken Satés with Coriander
Chicken with Coconut-Plum Sauce
Indian Tikka Chicken
Chicken with Indian Spices
Chicken Paprika
Chicken Adobo
Chicken Salad with Pesto and Fennel
Curried Chicken Salad with Cucumber
Burgundy Chicken
Breast of Duck with Red Wine Sauce

• Chicken with Lemon and Capers •

Tangy capers are a natural partner for chicken. In this dish the capers and lemon juice are mellowed when butter is whisked into the liquid, creating a rich sauce.

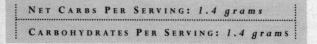

NET CARBS PER SERVING: *1.4 grams*

CARBOHYDRATES PER SERVING: *1.4 grams*

1 tablespoon olive oil
2 whole boneless chicken
    breasts, halved
75 ml white wine
1 tablespoon lemon juice

1 teaspoon grated lemon zest
1 tablespoon capers
25 g chilled butter, cut into
    small pieces

• Heat the oil in a heavy frying pan over a medium heat until hot but not smoking. Add the chicken and cook for 4 minutes on each side, or until browned. Remove the chicken from the frying pan and keep warm.

Add the wine, lemon juice, lemon zest and capers to the frying pan. Bring to the boil, lower the heat, and simmer for 2 minutes, making sure to scrape up any brown bits from the bottom of the frying pan. Whisk in the butter, 1 piece at a time, and cook over a low heat for 1 minute, or until heated through. Pour the sauce over the chicken and serve immediately.

Serves 2

· Coconut Chicken Satés · with Coriander

The coconut milk marinade makes these chicken satés, a popular Thai dish, tender and juicy. Peanut Dipping Sauce (page 174) is the traditional accompaniment.

> **NET CARBS PER SERVING:** *3.4 grams*
>
> **CARBOHYDRATES PER SERVING:** *3.5 grams*

one 400 ml can unsweetened coconut milk; reserve 1 tablespoon if making the Peanut Dipping Sauce

6 tablespoons chopped fresh coriander

1 teaspoon chopped fresh jalapeño pepper

1 small clove garlic, finely chopped

juice of ½ lime

salt and pepper to taste

2 whole boneless chicken breasts, cut into 2.5-cm strips

10 bamboo skewers, soaked in water for 30 minutes, or 10 metal skewers (see Note)

- Preheat the grill.

Combine the coconut milk, coriander, jalapeño, garlic, lime juice, salt and pepper in a large bowl and mix well. Add the chicken, stirring to coat. Let the chicken marinate, covered, in the refrigerator for at least 20 minutes or up to 1 hour.

Thread 2 pieces of chicken on to each skewer and grill, turning once, for 7 minutes, or until the chicken is lightly browned. Transfer to a serving plate and serve immediately.

Serves 2

Note: This dish can also be prepared without the skewers. Simply transfer the marinated strips to a grill pan and grill in the same manner.

• Chicken with •
Coconut-Plum Sauce

This lovely chicken dish features an unusual combination of flavours. You can double or triple the recipe for a great dinner party main course.

> **NET CARBS PER SERVING: 6.4 grams**
>
> **CARBOHYDRATES PER SERVING: 9.6 grams**

25 g butter

2 whole boneless chicken
   breasts, halved

250 ml unsweetened coconut
   milk

1 tablespoon Dijon mustard

1 teaspoon crumbled dried
   tarragon or 2 teaspoons
   chopped fresh tarragon

salt and pepper to taste

1 small plum, halved, stoned,
   and thinly sliced

3 tablespoons coarsely chopped
   almonds, lightly toasted
   (see Hint on page 172)

• Heat the butter in a large, deep frying pan over a medium-high heat until the foam subsides. Add the chicken and sauté for about 3 minutes on each side, until lightly browned. Add the coconut milk to the frying pan. Bring to a gentle boil, lower the heat, and simmer for 6 minutes, turning the chicken several times. Stir in the mustard, tarragon, salt, pepper and sliced plum, making sure to coat the chicken, and cook over a medium heat for 3 minutes. Remove from the heat and stir in the almonds. Serve immediately.

Serves 2

• Indian Tikka Chicken •

This simple recipe is absolutely delicious served with cucumber salad.

> **NET CARBS PER SERVING:** *1 gram*
>
> **CARBOHYDRATES PER SERVING:** *1 gram*

¾ cup whole milk yoghurt
1 tablespoon minced fresh
  gingerroot
1 tablespoon chopped cilantro
  plus additional for
  garnish
2 teaspoons chilli powder
1 teaspoon ground coriander

1 teaspoon dried mint
1 tablespoon olive oil
½ teaspoon salt
675 g skinless, boneless
  chicken breasts, cut into
  2.5-cm cubes
lime wedges for garnish

- In a shallow bowl combine the yoghurt, ginger, cilantro, chilli powder, coriander and mint and mix well. Add the chicken, cover, and marinate refrigerated for 4 hours and up to overnight.

About 1 hour before cooking, remove the chicken from refrigerator and bring to room temperature. Soak 4–6 thin wooden or bamboo skewers in water. Heat over to 375°F. Thread chicken on skewers, place on a baking sheet and drizzle with oil. Sprinkle with salt. Bake for 30 minutes, turning once halfway through cooking time, until golden brown and cooked through. Sprinkle with chopped cilantro and garnish with lime.

Serves 4

• Chicken with Indian Spices •

When simmered in turmeric, also known as Indian saffron, chicken breasts become wonderfully aromatic. Turmeric has been revered for centuries, not only for its flavour but also for its medicinal properties. Rich in potassium and vitamin C, turmeric acts as an excellent anti-inflammatory, according to traditional Indian medicine. The addition of soured cream makes this dish smooth and sumptuous.

NET CARBS PER SERVING: 6.1 grams
CARBOHYDRATES PER SERVING: 6.2 grams

45 g butter
1 whole boneless chicken
    breast, cut into strips
1½ teaspoons cumin
1½ teaspoons turmeric
¼ teaspoon dried hot chilli
    pepper flakes (optional)

4 cloves garlic, finely chopped
100 ml chicken stock
100 ml soured cream
1 tablespoon chopped fresh
    coriander or flat-leaf
    parsley for garnish
    (optional)

• Heat the butter in a heavy casserole over a medium-high heat until the foam subsides. Add the chicken strips and sauté, stirring, for about 2 minutes, until browned. Add the cumin, turmeric, chilli flakes and garlic, and sauté the mixture, stirring occasionally, for 2 minutes. Add the chicken stock and bring to the boil. Lower the heat to medium-low and simmer the mixture, stirring occasionally, for 10 minutes. Slowly add the soured cream and simmer the mixture (do not let it boil) for 3 minutes, or until heated through. Transfer the chicken with the sauce to a serving plate, garnish with the coriander or parsley if desired, and serve immediately.

Serves 2

• Chicken Paprika •

The first time I made this dish, Dr Atkins was effusive in his praise. I hope you will receive the same kudos when you serve it.

> NET CARBS PER SERVING: 9.1–4.6 grams
>
> CARBOHYDRATES PER SERVING: 10.2–5.1 grams

25 g butter
50 ml olive oil
150 g chopped onion
1 chicken (about 1.35 kg), cut
     into 8 to 12 pieces
1 tablespoon Hungarian
     paprika (available at
     specialty-food stores)

salt and pepper to taste
50 ml chicken stock
50 ml white wine
1 large egg yolk
100 ml soured cream

• Heat the butter and 2 tablespoons of oil in a frying pan over a medium-high heat until the foam subsides. Add the onion and sauté, stirring, for 3 minutes. Add the chicken pieces, skin side down, and sauté for 5 minutes on each side. Stir in the paprika, salt, pepper and the remaining olive oil. Cook, stirring, for about 2 minutes.

Meanwhile, bring the chicken stock and wine to the boil in a small saucepan. Whisk together the egg yolk and soured cream in a bowl. Slowly add the wine-stock mixture into the egg mixture, whisking until the sauce is smooth. Pour the sauce over the chicken in the frying pan, cover, and simmer for 10 minutes. Serve immediately.

Serves 2–4

• Chicken Adobo •

The tangy vinegar marinade called adobo is a Spanish influence on the cuisine of the Phillipines, and it goes beautifully with chicken.

> **NET CARBS PER SERVING: 6 grams**
>
> **CARBOHYDRATES PER SERVING: 6.5 grams**

1 cup white vinegar
2 cloves garlic, crushed
1 bay leaf
1½ teaspoons whole
    peppercorns, lightly
    crushed
½ cup reduced-sodium soy
    sauce

6 whole chicken legs, cut into
    drumstick and thigh
    pieces
1 cup water
3 tablespoons canola oil

• In a large glass baking dish, mix vinegar, garlic, bay leaf, peppercorns and soy sauce; add the chicken and toss to coat. Cover with plastic wrap and marinate in the refrigerator for 1 hour.

Transfer the chicken and its marinade to a large saucepan. Add water and heat to boiling over a high heat. Cover, reduce heat to low and simmer for 20 minutes. With tongs, transfer the chicken to a plate to cool. Boil cooking liquid until it is reduced to 1 cup for about 10 minutes. Let the sauce cool and strain into a small saucepan. Skim off fat and reheat.

Pat the chicken dry with paper towels. In a large frying pan, heat the oil over a high heat until very hot. Brown the chicken in batches for about 2 minutes per side. Transfer to a deep platter and pour hot sauce over chicken.

Serves 4

• Chicken Salad with Pesto • and Fennel

Fresh-tasting pesto and the liquorice-like flavour of fennel permeates this delicious and unusual chicken salad.

> NET CARBS PER SERVING: *3.8 grams*
>
> CARBOHYDRATES PER SERVING: *4.5 grams*

15 g butter
2 whole boneless chicken breasts, cut into 2.5-cm strips
juice of ½ lemon
3 tablespoons Basil Pesto (page 169)

1 small fennel bulb, halved lengthways, cored and thinly sliced
½ red pepper, chopped
salt and pepper to taste

• Heat the butter in a frying pan over a medium-high heat until the foam subsides. Add the chicken, drizzle it with the lemon juice, and sauté, turning frequently, for about 5 minutes, until golden. Stir in 2 tablespoons of pesto, coating the chicken well.

Transfer the chicken to a large serving bowl. Add the fennel, red pepper, salt, pepper and remaining pesto, and toss the salad well. Serve immediately or store, covered, in the refrigerator for up to 1 day.

Serves 2

• Curried Chicken Salad •
with Cucumber

The sweet and spicy flavour of curry powder contrasts with the coolness of cucumber in this aromatic salad. A touch of cinnamon adds a hint of intrigue.

> **NET CARBS PER SERVING: 3.1 grams**
>
> **CARBOHYDRATES PER SERVING: 4.2 grams**

100 ml mayonnaise
1 teaspoon curry powder
½ teaspoon cinnamon
1 tablespoon grated onion
1 tablespoon chopped fresh
    flat-leaf parsley

1 teaspoon balsamic vinegar
salt and pepper to taste
350 g cubed cooked chicken
1 stick celery, chopped
85 g chopped, seeded and
    peeled cucumber

• Whisk together the mayonnaise, curry powder, cinnamon, onion, parsley, vinegar, salt and pepper in a large serving bowl. Add the chicken, celery and cucumber, and toss the salad well. Serve immediately or store, covered, in the refrigerator for up to 1 day.

Serves 2

• Burgundy Chicken •

This favourite winter warmer is more of a braise than a stew because there is very little cooking liquid. The wine imparts a rich flavour, but almost all of the alcohol evaporates as the dish simmers.

> **NET CARBS PER SERVING: 3 grams**
>
> **CARBOHYDRATES PER SERVING: 3.5 grams**

2 tablespoons olive oil,
    divided
1 small onion, chopped
½ small carrot, chopped
1 celery stalk, chopped
2 cloves garlic, sliced
50 g baked ham, diced
900 g boneless, skinless
    chicken thighs

½ cup red wine
½ cup reduced-sodium chicken
    broth
½ bay leaf
2 tablespoons chopped fresh
    parsley

• Heat 1 tablespoon oil in a large, heavy frying pan over a medium heat. Add the onion, carrot and celery. Cook for 5 minutes, until the vegetables soften. Add the garlic and ham and cook for 2 minutes more. Transfer the mixture to a bowl.

Heat the remaining oil and brown the chicken thighs. Add the wine, broth and bay leaf to the pan. Reduce heat to medium-low and cook for 35 minutes, until the chicken is cooked through and most of the liquid has reduced. Return the vegetables and ham to the pan. Mix well and heat through for 5 minutes. Sprinkle with parsley before serving.

Serves 4

· Breast of Duck with ·
Red Wine Sauce

Sliced duck drizzled with a rich wine sauce makes a sophisticated main course for a formal dinner. The recipe can be doubled or tripled according to the number of guests. Serve with Green Beans with Anchovy Sauce (page 151).

> NET CARBS PER SERVING: *6.3 grams*
>
> CARBOHYDRATES PER SERVING: *6.5 grams*

1 whole boneless duck breast
15 g butter
1 large shallot, finely chopped
100 ml dry red wine
1 tablespoon balsamic vinegar

1 tablespoon soy sauce
1 tablespoon Worcestershire
  sauce
1 beef bouillon cube
50 ml double cream

• **Prick the duck all over with a fork. Heat a nonstick frying pan over a medium-high heat until hot. Place the duck, skin side down, in the frying pan and cook for 8 to 10 minutes, or until the skin is crisp and brown. Turn the duck and cook for another 5 minutes. Remove the duck from the frying pan and keep warm.**

Heat the butter in the frying pan over a medium heat until the foam subsides. Add the shallot and cook for about 1 minute, until barely golden. Add the wine, vinegar, soy sauce, Worcestershire sauce and bouillon cube. Bring to the boil, lower the heat, and simmer for 5 minutes. Add the cream and cook over a medium heat, stirring occasionally, for 2 minutes, or until the sauce is heated through (do not let it boil). Cut the duck into thin slices, arrange them on 2 plates, and top with sauce. Serve immediately.

Serves 2

Pork

•

Stir-Fried Pork with Water Chestnuts
Mustard-Crusted Pork
Pork Chops with Orange and Rosemary
Pork with Chilli Sauce
Peppery Pork Chops
Garlic Dill Meatballs
Barbecued Spareribs

• Stir-Fried Pork with •
Water Chestnuts

Crunchy water chestnuts add a wonderful texture to this simple stir-fry with delicious Asian flavours.

> **NET CARBS PER SERVING: 5.4 grams**
>
> **CARBOHYDRATES PER SERVING: 7.1 grams**

450 g pork loin
2 tablespoons rapeseed oil
75 g chopped onion
½ tablespoon peeled and finely
    chopped gingerroot
3 cloves garlic, finely chopped
75 g sliced water chestnuts

25 g sliced mushrooms
1 tablespoon dry white wine
salt and pepper to taste
1 tablespoon toasted sesame
    oil
1 tablespoon soy sauce

• Cut the pork into 5 mm slices and then into thin strips.

Heat the oil in a large, heavy frying pan or a wok over a medium-high heat until hot but not smoking. Add the pork and stir-fry for 3 to 4 minutes, or until the pork begins to brown. Add the onion, gingerroot and garlic, and stir-fry for 1 minute. Add the water chestnuts and mushrooms, and stir-fry for 2 minutes. Add the wine, salt, pepper, sesame oil and soy sauce, and stir-fry for 2 minutes. Serve immediately.

Serves 2

• Mustard-Crusted Pork •

Tofu flour works as a wonderful alternative for dusting and dredging your foods. It also provides the health benefits of soya without the nutritional pitfalls of overprocessed bleached white flour. Serve with Horseradish Cream (page 177).

> NET CARBS PER SERVING: *1.1 grams*
>
> CARBOHYDRATES PER SERVING: *2.7 grams*

2 tablespoons tofu flour or
    soya flour (available at
    some natural-food stores)
1 tablespoon mustard powder
½ teaspoon white pepper
50 ml olive oil

450 g boneless pork loin, cut
    against the grain into 3
    strips (about 1-cm thick)
salt to taste

• **Combine the tofu flour, mustard powder and pepper in a bowl and mix well. Dust the pork with the flour mixture. Heat 2 tablespoons of the oil in a heavy frying pan over a medium heat until hot but not smoking. Add half of the pork (do not crowd the frying pan) and brown for 5 minutes on each side, or until cooked through. Repeat with the remaining oil and pork. Sprinkle the pork with salt and serve immediately.**

Serves 2

• Pork Chops with Orange • and Rosemary

In this recipe, orange and mustard enliven the flavour of meaty pork chops. The sauce is so sweet and tangy that you'll never miss the traditional apple sauce.

> NET CARBS PER SERVING: *4 grams*
>
> CARBOHYDRATES PER SERVING: *5.1 grams*

2 loin or chump pork chops
    (each about 2-cm thick)
salt and pepper to taste
soya flour, tofu flour or whey
    protein (all available at
    natural-food stores) for
    dusting the pork chops
25 g butter, plus an extra
    knob for frying the
    shallots
3 tablespoons chopped shallots

75 ml dry white wine
1 teaspoon tomato purée
1 teaspoon Worcestershire
    sauce
1 tablespoon grated orange
    zest
1 teaspoon Dijon mustard
3/4 teaspoon crumbled dried
    rosemary or 1 1/2
    teaspoons chopped fresh
    rosemary

• Season the pork chops with salt and pepper, and lightly dust with soya flour, shaking off any excess. Heat the 25 g of butter in a frying pan over a medium-high heat until the foam subsides and sauté the pork chops for 5 minutes on each side. Transfer the pork chops to a serving plate and keep warm.

Heat the remaining butter until the foam subsides and sauté the shallots for about 30 seconds, until softened. Add the wine, tomato purée, Worcestershire sauce, orange zest, mustard and rosemary to the frying pan. Bring to the boil, lower the heat, and simmer the sauce for 2 minutes, making sure to scrape up any brown bits from the bottom of the frying pan. Pour the sauce over the pork chops and serve immediately.

Serves 2

• Pork with Chilli Sauce •

Serrano chilli gives this dish a wonderful southwestern flavour.
You can use beef instead of pork for a delicious variation.

> **NET CARBS PER SERVING: 7.8 grams**
>
> **CARBOHYDRATES PER SERVING: 8.7 grams**

1 spring onion (including ¾
   of the green part),
   chopped
3 cloves garlic
45 g chopped green pepper
75 g chopped fresh or canned
   tomatillos (available at
   specialty food stores) or
   red or green tomato

1 serrano chilli or jalapeño
   pepper, seeded and
   chopped
100 ml beef stock
1 tablespoon fresh lime juice
2 tablespoons dry sherry
675 g pork loin, cubed
1 tablespoon paprika
3 tablespoons olive oil

• **Preheat the grill.**

Combine the spring onion, garlic, green pepper, tomatillos, chilli, beef stock, lime juice and sherry in a food processor and process for 1 minute, or until well blended. Transfer the mixture to a saucepan, bring to a boil, lower the heat, and simmer for 10 minutes.

Meanwhile, place the pork in a grill pan, sprinkle with paprika and oil, and grill for 8 to 10 minutes, turning the pork to brown on all sides. Transfer the pork to a serving plate and pour the chilli sauce over it. Serve immediately.

Serves 2

• Peppery Pork Chops •

The Mexican flavours complement the rich pork flavour, and marinating the chops makes them even more tender. This one is always popular.

> **NET CARBS PER SERVING:** *3.4 grams*
>
> **CARBOHYDRATES PER SERVING:** *3.5 grams*

4 boneless pork loin chops (175 g), about 2.5-cm thick

1 tin (125 g) chopped green chillies

½ chipotle en adobo*, chopped

2 garlic cloves, minced

1 tablespoon dried oregano

2 teaspoons ground cumin

¼ cup cider vinegar

1 packet sugar substitute (do not use Equal or aspartame; they lose their sweetness when heated)

1 tablespoon canola oil

• Combine the chillies, garlic, oregano, cumin and vinegar in a blender and purée. Place the pork chops in a shallow baking dish and pour the pepper mixture on top. Turn the chops to coat. Marinate for 4–8 hours.

Drain the pork chops and pat dry. Place marinade in a small saucepan. Mix in sugar substitute, bring to the boil; cook for 3 minutes.

Heat the oil in a large frying pan and cook the chops for 10 minutes, turning once halfway through cooking time, just until cooked through. Serve with the cooked marinade.

Serves 4

* Chipotles en adobo are smoked jalapenos in a spicy tomato sauce. They are hot so add less if you prefer a milder dish. They come in small cans, and last forever in the fridge if transferred to a covered glass or plastic container.

• Garlic Dill Meatballs •

Ever since I prepared this dish for a dinner party, I've been getting requests for an encore. Serve the meatballs alone on cocktail sticks as an hors d'oeuvre or on a layer of Creamy Mushroom Sauce (page 179) as a main course or first course. You can double or triple the recipe as needed.

> NET CARBS: *1 gram per meatball*
>
> CARBOHYDRATES: *1 gram per meatball*

450 g minced chicken
450 g minced pork
1 small onion, finely chopped
75 g minced pork rinds
    (optional)
1 large egg

2 cloves garlic, finely
    choppped
2 tablespoons chopped fresh
    dill
salt and pepper to taste
2 tablespoons rapeseed oil

* Preheat the oven to 190°C/375°F, gas mark 5.

Combine the chicken, pork, onion, pork rinds, if using, egg, garlic, dill, salt and pepper in a bowl and mix well. Divide the mixture into twelve 5-cm meatballs.

Heat the oil in a large ovenproof frying pan over a medium-high heat until hot but not smoking. Brown the meatballs, turning them, for about 6 minutes. Transfer the frying pan to the oven and bake the meatballs, covered, for 15 minutes. Serve immediately.

Makes about 12 meatballs

• Barbecued Spareribs •

Ribs are one of my favourite indulgences on the Atkins diet. I have created a quick version that you can make even after a long day at work.

> NET CARBS PER SERVING: 0.9 gram
>
> CARBOHYDRATES PER SERVING: 1 gram

1.35 kg spareribs
2 bay leaves
2 tablespoons whole
    peppercorns
45 g butter, softened
1 tablespoon unsweetened

ketchup (available at
specialty-food stores and
some supermarkets)
2 teaspoons hot chilli pepper
sauce

• Preheat the grill.

Place the ribs in a large pot, cover with water, and add the bay leaves and peppercorns. Bring to the boil, lower the heat, cover, and simmer for 20 minutes.

Meanwhile, combine the butter, ketchup and chilli sauce in a small bowl. Drain the ribs. Pat the butter mixture on all sides of the ribs and grill them for 2 to 3 minutes on each side, or until browned and crisp. Serve immediately.

Serves 2

Lamb

●

Grilled Marinated Lamb Chops
Grilled Lemon and Rosemary Lamb
Shortcut Moussaka

• Grilled Marinated Lamb Chops •

Simple and scrumptious, these lamb chops burst with the zesty flavour of the marinade, which also gives them a wonderful glazelike crust. Serve with Red Pepper Purée (page 167).

> NET CARBS PER SERVING: *1.3 grams*
>
> CARBOHYDRATES PER SERVING: *1.4 grams*

2 tablespoons olive oil
1 tablespoon Worcestershire
   sauce
2 tablespoons lime juice
2 tablespoons soy sauce

2 tablespoons dry white wine
3 cloves garlic, finely chopped
salt and pepper to taste
450 g lamb chops (each about
   2-cm thick)

- Preheat the grill.

Whisk together the oil, Worcestershire sauce, lime juice, soy sauce, wine, garlic, salt and pepper in a large bowl. Add the lamb chops and let them marinate, covered, in the refrigerator for 15 minutes or up to 1 hour.

Remove the lamb chops from the marinade and pat dry. Grill the lamb chops for 4 minutes on each side for medium-rare, or until desired doneness. Serve immediately.

Serves 2

• Grilled Lemon and •
Rosemary Lamb

Lamb is one of Dr Atkins' favourite dishes, and this rendition could not be simpler. The marinade coats each piece of lamb, making it succulent and flavoursome.

> NET CARBS PER SERVING: 3.7 grams
>
> CARBOHYDRATES PER SERVING: 3.8 grams

5 tablespoons fresh lemon
   juice
100 ml olive oil
1 tablespoon fresh rosemary or
   1½ teaspoons dried
   rosemary

1 clove garlic, finely chopped
2 teaspoons grated lemon zest
450 g boneless lamb chops, cut
   into 2.5-cm cubes

• Preheat the griddle.

Whisk together the lemon juice, oil, rosemary, garlic and lemon zest in a bowl. Add the lamb and toss gently, making sure each piece is well coated. Cover and put in the refrigerator for 10 to 15 minutes. Thread the lamb on to skewers and grill, turning once, for 12 minutes for medium. Serve immediately.

Serves 2

• Shortcut Moussaka •

Moussaka is a delicious one-dish-meal and wonderful on chilly nights. The trouble is that it used to take hours to prepare. Our low carb version is a lot faster than traditional recipes, but just as good.

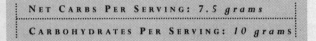

NET CARBS PER SERVING: 7.5 grams

CARBOHYDRATES PER SERVING: 10 grams

3 tablespoons olive oil,
    divided
½ small onion, chopped
2 cloves garlic, chopped
700 g lean ground lamb
½ cup red wine
1 tablespoon tomato paste
1 cup carbohydrate controlled
    tomato sauce
½ teaspoon salt

¼ teaspoon ground cinnamon
dash of ground cloves
1 medium aubergine, peeled
    and sliced diagonally in
    0.5-cm slices
175 g cream cheese
¼ cup cream
¼ teaspoon nutmeg
¼ cup grated feta cheese

• **Preheat the oven to 425°F. Heat 1 tablespoon of the oil in a large pan over a medium heat. Cook the onion for 3 minutes until soft; add garlic and lamb. Cook the lamb for 5 minutes, until no longer pink, breaking up with a wooden spoon. Drain off the fat; stir in the wine, tomato paste, tomato sauce, salt, cinnamon, and cloves. Bring to the boil; reduce heat to low and simmer 10 minutes.**

While the sauce is cooking, prepare the aubergine. Brush slices with the remaining oil. Arrange in a single layer on a baking sheet and bake for 12 to 15 minutes until lightly browned and softened. Flip slices halfway through cooking time.

In a small saucepan, cook the cream cheese, cream and nutmeg just until the cream cheese melts; whisk until smooth. Set aside.

Reduce oven temperature to 350°F. Oil a 22-cm square baking pan and spread a thin layer of meat sauce on bottom. Layer half the aubergine slices on top; cover with half the remaining meat sauce and half the cream sauce. Repeat layers. Sprinkle with feta cheese. Bake for 20 minutes until the cheese starts to brown. Serve hot or at room temperature.

Serves 6

Beef

•

Spiced Steak

Filets Mignons with Zesty Wine Sauce

Rib-eye Steak with Red Wine Sauce

Grilled Steaks with Mustard-Herb Rub

Sirloin Steak with Cognac Mustard Sauce

Lemon-Thyme Tenderloin with Roasted Vegetables

Beef Burgers with Feta and Tomato

Chevapchichi (Spicy Meat Rolls)

Burrito Beef

Chilli Beef Kebabs

Burgundy Beef Stew

Asian Beef Salad

• Spiced Steak •

Simple and flavoursome, this quick-to-fix steak is a great staple for the Atkins eating plan. Serve it with Roasted Peppers in Garlic Oil (page 157) or try tossing the sliced steak with baby greens and your favourite homemade dressing.

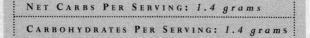

NET CARBS PER SERVING: *1.4 grams*

CARBOHYDRATES PER SERVING: *1.4 grams*

1 teaspoon paprika
1 teaspoon cumin
1 teaspoon ground coriander

salt and pepper to taste
450 g steak (sirloin, fillet or rump)

● **Preheat the grill.**

Combine the paprika, cumin, coriander, salt and pepper in a small bowl. Rub the spice mixture over the entire surface of the steak and let the steak marinate, covered with cling film, in the refrigerator for 20 minutes.

Grill the steak for 2½ to 3 minutes on each side for medium-rare. Let stand for 5 minutes.

Cut the steak diagonally into thin slices. Serve immediately or store in the refrigerator, wrapped well, for up to 2 days.

Serves 2

• Filets Mignons with •
Zesty Wine Sauce

Filets mignons make the perfect elegant dinner for two. In this recipe the zestiness of the red wine sauce contrasts beautifully with the tender beef. Serve Fennel Salad with Parmesan (page 64) as a starter.

> NET CARBS PER SERVING: 4.6 grams
>
> CARBOHYDRATES PER SERVING: 4.7 grams

250 ml dry red wine
juice of 1 lime
60 ml olive oil
3 cloves garlic, finely chopped
1/2 teaspoon freshly ground
   pepper
100 ml beef stock

4 filets mignons (each about
   2-cm thick)
25 g butter
4 oil-packed anchovy fillets,
   mashed
2 tablespoons soured cream

• Whisk together the wine, lime juice, all but 1 tablespoon of the oil, the garlic, pepper and beef stock in a large bowl. Add the filets mignons to the marinade and let stand for 10 minutes. Heat the butter and remaining tablespoon of oil in a heavy frying pan over a medium-high heat until hot but not smoking. Remove the filets from the marinade and pat dry. Reserve the marinade. Sauté the filets for 4 minutes on each side for medium-rare. Transfer the filets to a plate and keep warm.

Add the reserved marinade and anchovies to the frying pan and boil, stirring frequently, for 5 minutes. Whisk in the soured cream and cook over a low heat for 2 minutes, or until the sauce is heated through (do not let it boil). Pour the sauce over the filets and serve immediately.

Serves 2

• Rib-eye Steak with •
Red Wine Sauce

This rich, comforting dish is perfect for the colder months. If you have access to fresh herbs, add some chopped tarragon or rosemary to the sauce.

> **NET CARBS PER SERVING:** *1 gram*
>
> **CARBOHYDRATES PER SERVING:** *1.5 grams*

2 tablespoons olive oil
450 g boneless rib-eye steak
    (about 1-cm thick)
15 g butter
2 large cloves garlic, finely
    chopped

3 tablespoons shallots, finely
    chopped
100 ml red wine
50 ml beef stock
¼ teaspoon freshly ground
    pepper
salt to taste

• Heat the oil in a large, heavy frying pan over a medium-high heat until hot but not smoking. Lower the heat to medium, add the steak, and cook for 6 minutes on each side for medium. Remove the steak from the frying pan and keep warm.

Heat the butter in the frying pan until the foam subsides. Add the garlic and shallots, and cook, stirring, for 3 minutes, or until the shallots become transparent. Add the wine, stock, pepper and salt. Bring to the boil, making sure to scrape up any brown bits from the bottom of the frying pan. Lower the heat and simmer for 3 minutes. Slice the steak into thin strips and top with the wine sauce. Serve immediately.

Serves 2

• Grilled Steaks with •
Mustard-Herb Rub

If you enjoy the flavour of mustard, try this rub (it is also delicious on grilled pork chops).

> NET CARBS PER SERVING: *1.5 grams*
>
> CARBOHYDRATES PER SERVING: *2 grams*

2 tablespoons Dijon style
    mustard
2 large garlic cloves, crushed
½ teaspoon crumbled dried
    rosemary leaves
½ teaspoon dried thyme leaves

½ teaspoon dried oregano
½ teaspoon pepper
4 trimmed beef rib eye or
    boneless top loin steaks,
    2.5-cm thick
salt

• **Combine the mustard, garlic, rosemary, thyme, oregano and pepper. Spread the mixture on both sides of the steaks.**

Grill the steaks over medium hot coals, turning occasionally. Cook for 11 to 14 minutes for medium-rare to medium (if using top loin steaks, grill a little longer), turning halfway through cooking time. Season with salt to taste.

Serves 4

· Sirloin Steak with ·
Cognac Mustard Sauce

This elegant dish can be prepared in only fifteen minutes. It makes the perfect romantic dinner main course for two.

> NET CARBS PER SERVING: *4.3 grams*
>
> CARBOHYDRATES PER SERVING: *4.3 grams*

675 g boneless sirloin steak
    (about 1-cm thick)
50 g butter
50 ml double cream
3 tablespoons Cognac

1 tablespoon Dijon mustard
2 tablespoons Worcestershire
    sauce
salt and pepper to taste

• Cut the steak into 4 pieces. Place each piece between 2 sheets of cling film and pound until thin, about 3 mm thick. Heat half the butter in a large, heavy frying pan over a medium-high heat until the foam subsides. Sauté the steak, in batches if necessary (do not crowd the frying pan), for about 45 seconds on each side. Transfer the steak to a serving plate and keep warm.

Add the remaining butter, cream, Cognac, mustard, Worcestershire sauce, salt and pepper to the frying pan. Bring to the boil, lower the heat, and simmer the sauce for 3 minutes, making sure to scrape up any brown bits from the bottom of the frying pan. Pour the sauce over the steak and serve immediately.

Serves 2

• Lemon-Thyme Tenderloin •
with Roasted Vegetables

Sweet peppers and green onions surround lemon-and-thyme-seasoned beef tenderloin in this elegant entrée.

> NET CARBS PER SERVING: *2.5 grams*
>
> CARBOHYDRATES PER SERVING: *4 grams*

3 tablespoons olive oil

2 tablespoons grated lemon peel

2 teaspoons dried thyme leaves

1 teaspoon dried marjoram

1½ teaspoons salt

1 teaspoon pepper

1 beef tenderloin roast (1.8 kilos), trimmed

1 small red pepper, cut into 2.5-cm wedges

1 small yellow pepper, cut into 2.5-cm wedges

8 spring onions, cut into 2-cm pieces

2 yellow squash, cut into 2.5-cm pieces

• Heat the oven to 425°F. Combine the lemon, oil, thyme, marjoram, salt and pepper in a bowl; rub half the mixture over tenderloin and toss remaining mixture with the vegetables to coat.

Place the beef in a large roasting pan and roast for 40 minutes. Add the vegetables to the pan. Continue cooking until a meat thermometer inserted in the tenderloin registers 135°F for medium rare or 145°F for medium doneness.

Transfer the roast to a cutting board and let rest for 5 minutes before slicing.

Serves 8

• Beef Burgers with •
Feta and Tomato

Think of these burgers as mini meatloaves with lots of flavours. They are great grilled and equally delicious panfried. Serve with Creamy Celery Sauce (page 176) or Cucumber-Dill Sauce (page 175).

> NET CARBS PER SERVING: *2 grams*
>
> CARBOHYDRATES PER SERVING: *2.5 grams*

450 g minced beef (silverside or topside)
1 1/2 teaspoons chopped fresh thyme leaves or 3/4 teaspoon crumbled dried thyme
1 spring onion (white part only), chopped
50 g chopped fresh spinach
50 g chopped tomato
50 g crumbled feta cheese
salt and pepper to taste
1 teaspoon chopped fresh mint leaves (optional)

• Combine the minced beef, thyme, spring onion, spinach, tomato, feta, salt, pepper and mint, if desired, in a large bowl and mix well. Form into 2 patties. Grill or panfry over a medium-high heat for 5 minutes on each side for medium-rare, or until desired doneness. Serve immediately.

Serves 2

• Chevapchichi (Spicy Meat Rolls) •

They're not your mother's meatballs. Flavoursome and rich, these hot and spicy meat rolls pair nicely with our refreshing chilled Cucumber-Dill Sauce (page 175).

> **NET CARBS PER SERVING: 5.2 grams**
>
> **CARBOHYDRATES PER SERVING: 5.8 grams**

225 g minced veal
225 g minced beef
225 g minced pork
2 tablespoons soda water
½ medium onion, finely
chopped
2 cloves garlic, finely chopped
1 tablespoon finely chopped
fresh flat-leaf parsley

1 teaspoon Hungarian
paprika
½ teaspoon freshly ground
pepper
2 tablespoons olive oil
salt to taste

• Combine the veal, beef, pork, soda water, onion, garlic, parsley, paprika and pepper in a large bowl and mix well. Take 1 heaped tablespoon of the mixture and shape it into a 7–8-cm roll. Continue making rolls in the same manner until all the mixture is used. (You will have 15 to 20 rolls.)

Heat the oil in a heavy frying pan over a medium heat until it is hot but not smoking. Cook the rolls in batches, turning them frequently, about 12 to 15 minutes, until nicely browned. Sprinkle the rolls with salt and serve immediately.

Serves 2—4

• Burrito Beef •

To make a complete meal, roll shredded beef in controlled carbohydrate tortillas and top with sour cream, chopped spring onions and salsa.

> NET CARBS PER SERVING: *2 grams*
>
> CARBOHYDRATES PER SERVING: *2.5 grams*

900 g boneless beef chuck
¼ cup green salsa
2 garlic cloves, crushed
2 spring onions, chopped
1 jalapeño pepper, seeded and
    chopped

2 teaspoons chilli powder
½ teaspoon ground cumin
½ teaspoon salt

- Trim the fat off the beef. Place the beef, salsa, garlic, spring onions, jalapeño, chilli powder, cumin and salt in slow cooker. Cover and cook on low for 8 hours until the beef is very tender.

    Remove the beef, and shred it with two forks. Mix the beef with ½ cup of cooking juices before filling the tortillas.

Serves 6

• Chilli Beef Kebabs •

Grilling brings out the best flavour in these tender cubes of beef.
Instead of onions, we used scallions, which are lower in carbs, in
our kebabs.

2 tablespoons canola oil
2 large garlic cloves, crushed
1 tablespoon chilli powder
a dash of ground red pepper
900 g boneless beef top sirloin,
    cut into 2.5-cm pieces

8 spring onions, cut into 2-cm
    pieces
2 tablespoons chopped fresh
    parsley

• **Combine the oil, garlic, chilli powder and red pepper in a
bowl. Add the beef and spring onions, tossing them in the marinade
until they're coated. Marinate for 20 minutes.**

**Prepare a medium heat grill. On eight 12-inch metal skewers,
alternately thread beef and green onion pieces. Grill the kebabs
for 10 to 12 minutes, turning occasionally, for medium-rare to
medium doneness. Season to taste with salt and then sprinkle
them with parsley.**

Serves 4

• Burgundy Beef Stew •

The technique of reducing the wine before adding the beef allows for almost all the alcohol to burn off and produce a very rich tasting sauce.

> NET CARBS PER SERVING: *6.9 grams*
>
> CARBOHYDRATES PER SERVING: *9.1 grams*

½ cup Atkins Bake Mix*
1.350 kg beef chuck or round, cut into 4-cm cubes
125 g sliced bacon
1 tablespoon oil
1 medium onion, chopped
1 carrot, chopped
1 celery stalk, chopped
2 garlic cloves, crushed

2 cups dry red wine
1 tin (400 g) reduced sodium beef broth plus 1 tin of water
1 bay leaf
1 teaspoon dried thyme
1 tablespoon butter
225 g button mushrooms

• Spread the bake mix in a shallow plate; dredge beef pieces, tap off the excess. In a large Dutch oven over a medium heat, cook the bacon until it's crisp. Remove the bacon, crumble it up and set aside.

Add the oil to the bacon fat in the Dutch oven. Brown the beef in batches and transfer to a platter. Add the onion, carrot and celery to the Dutch oven; cook for 8 minutes, until softened. Pour in the wine, increasing the heat to high. Boil the wine until it's reduced to 1 cup, which should take about 5 minutes.

Return beef and all the accumulated juices to the Dutch oven. Pour in the beef broth and water; add the bay leaf and thyme. Reduce the heat to low, cover partially and simmer for 1 hour, until the beef is tender.

Melt the butter in a large fyring pan over medium heat. Sauté the mushrooms until they're golden, which takes about 5 minutes. Add the mushrooms to the stew, along with the reserved bacon. Remove the bay leaf.

* Available from www.atkinscenter.com

Serves 6

· Asian Beef Salad ·

One simple and scrumptious sauce does double duty: as a marinade and then as a dressing to toss with salad greens.

NET CARBS PER SERVING: 6 grams

CARBOHYDRATES PER SERVING: 10.5 grams

Marinade and Dressing Base:
4 spring onions, chopped
3 garlic cloves, crushed
¼ cup soy sauce
2 tablespoons rice wine
    vinegar
2 teaspoons sesame oil
1 packet sugar substitute (do
    not use Equal or
    aspartame; they lose
    their sweetness when
    heated)

½ teaspoon curry powder
¼ teaspoon dried ginger
Salad Ingredients:
1½ pounds beef sirloin steak,
    cut against the grain
    into 0.4-cm strips
2 tablespoons canola oil
6 cups mixed salad greens
1 red pepper, thinly sliced
1 tin (225 g) sliced water
    chestnuts, drained

• Mix the green onions, garlic, soy sauce, rice wine vinegar, sesame oil and sugar substitute in a small bowl. Pour half the mixture into a re-sealable plastic bag; add the steak strips. To the remaining soy sauce mixture, add the curry powder and the ginger.

Heat the canola oil in a large frying pan over high heat until it's very hot. Drain the beef and discard the marinade; quickly stir-fry for 2 to 3 minutes in hot oil for medium doneness. Transfer the beef to a large mixing bowl.

Add the salad greens, pepper, water chestnuts and soy dressing. Toss to coat the salad in dressing.

Serves 4

Vegetables

•

Cauliflower with Cumin Seeds

Grilled Aubergine with Mint Sauce

Grilled Leeks with Lemon Vinaigrette

Sautéed Courgettes with Nutmeg

Baked Fennel au Gratin

Green Beans with Garlic-Tarragon Vinaigrette

Mangetout with Hazelnuts

Green Beans with Anchovy Sauce

Green Bean, Smoked Mozzarella and Tomato Salad

Sprouting Broccoli with Spicy Sausage

Green Beans with Sun-Dried Tomatoes
and Goat's Cheese

Sautéed Spinach with Garlic and Olive Oil

Puréed Avocado with Garlic and Tarragon

Roasted Peppers in Garlic Oil

Vegetable Medley

Stir-Fried Vegetables with Mustard Seeds
and Balsamic Vinegar

Stir-Fried Asparagus with Basil

Spinach and Cheddar Casserole

Sesame Broccoli, Red Pepper and Spinach

Tomato-Cucumber Guacamole

• Cauliflower with Cumin Seeds •

This fragrant dish can be served either hot or at room temperature.
If you are not a fan of cumin seeds, you can substitute an equal
amount of fennel or caraway seeds.

> NET CARBS PER SERVING: *4.3 grams*
>
> CARBOHYDRATES PER SERVING: *8.1 grams*

2 tablespoons cumin seeds
50 ml olive oil
2 cloves garlic, thinly sliced

1 large cauliflower, broken
  into florets, and cut into
  bite-sized pieces
salt and pepper to taste

• Heat a frying pan over a medium heat until hot but not
smoking. Add the cumin seeds and cook until the seeds begin to
brown and pop, about 1 minute. Remove from the frying pan and
reserve. Heat the oil in the same frying pan, add the garlic, and
sauté for 30 seconds. Add the cauliflower and sauté, stirring
occasionally, for about 5 minutes, until the cauliflower begins to
brown. Add the toasted cumin seeds, salt and pepper, toss well,
and serve.

Serves 2

• Grilled Aubergine •
with Mint Sauce

Smoky aubergine topped with a cool, garlicky-mint sauce makes a terrific first course or tasty side dish that pairs beautifully with chicken or lamb.

> NET CARBS PER SERVING: 7.5 grams
>
> CARBOHYDRATES PER SERVING: 11.5 grams

¾ cup whole-milk yoghurt
2 tablespoons sour cream
½ cup freshly chopped mint
4 spring onions, chopped
¼ teaspoon salt
⅛ teaspoon ground pepper
1 large garlic clove, crushed

¼ cup olive oil
2 medium aubergines (about 900 grams), cut in 1-cm slices
1 large garlic clove, halved
½ teaspoon salt
¼ teaspoon ground pepper

• In a medium bowl, mix the yoghurt, sour cream, mint, onions, salt, pepper and garlic until the ingredients are well combined. Refrigerate the mixture while you grill the aubergine, for the flavours to blend.

Prepare a medium grill; brush with a little olive oil. Rub both sides of the aubergine slices with garlic and brush with the remaining oil. Sprinkle with salt and pepper.

Grill the aubergine for 20 to 25 minutes or until tender, turning halfway through the cooking time. Serve with the mint sauce.

Serves 6

• Grilled Leeks with Lemon •
Vinaigrette

Sweet, fragrant leeks are a must to try on the grill because their flavour intensifies. Be sure to wash them well though to remove all the dirt.

> NET CARBS PER SERVING: *8 grams*
>
> CARBOHYDRATES PER SERVING: *9.5 grams*

About 900 g leeks, trimmed
    and cleaned, split
    lengthwise if large
2 tablespoons extra virgin
    olive oil

1 teaspoon chopped fresh
    rosemary
salt and freshly ground pepper
¼ cup lemon vinaigrette

• **Prepare a hot grill. Brush the leeks with the oil and sprinkle with rosemary, salt and pepper.**

Grill directly on the rack or place in a grill basket and cook, turning occasionally, until the leeks are very tender, for 10 to 15 minutes, depending on their thickness. Transfer to a serving platter and drizzle with the vinaigrette.

Serves 6

• Sautéed Courgettes with Nutmeg •

The delicacy of this speedy sauté makes it a perfect partner for
Mustard-Crusted Pork (page 117).

> NET CARBS PER SERVING: 3.7 grams
>
> CARBOHYDRATES PER SERVING: 3.9 grams

25 g butter
2 medium courgettes, cut into
   1-cm-thick slices

salt and pepper to taste
nutmeg to taste

- Heat the butter in a frying pan over a medium–high heat until
the foam subsides. Add the courgettes, and sauté for 10 minutes,
stirring frequently. Sprinkle with salt, pepper and nutmeg. Serve
immediately.

Serves 2

• Baked Fennel au Gratin •

The mild liquorice taste of fennel goes beautifully with cheese.

> NET CARBS PER SERVING: *8 grams*
>
> CARBOHYDRATES PER SERVING: *13 grams*

2 (450 g) fennel bulbs
½ teaspoon salt
¼ teaspoon pepper
½ stick unsalted butter, plus 1
    teaspoon
3 tablespoons Atkins Bake
    Mix*

1 cup cream
½ cup (125 grams) shredded
    Gruyère or Swiss cheese
2 tablespoons Parmesan cheese

• Heat your oven to 375°F. Trim the fennel leaving 2.5-cm stalks. Quarter the fennel bulbs, removing the central core and cut them crosswise into 1-cm slices. Place the fennel in a saucepan, adding ½ cup water, and cook over a medium heat for 10 minutes, until it's just tender. Drain the fennel and sprinkle it with salt and pepper.

Grease a shallow 2-litre baking dish with 1 teaspoon of butter. Transfer the fennel to the dish, pressing down to form an even layer.

In a medium saucepan melt the butter. Stir in the bake mix and cook for 2 minutes. Pour in the cream. Bring to the boil and cook for 5 minutes until slightly thickened. Add the Gruyère cheese and stir until it's melted. Pour the sauce evenly over the fennel. Sprinkle the dish with Parmesan cheese.

Cover with foil and bake for 15 minutes, uncover and bake for a further 15 minutes until it's golden brown and bubbly.

Serves 6

* Available from www.atkinscenter.com

• Green Beans with •
Garlic-Tarragon Vinaigrette

Green beans are wonderfully flavoursome when they are tossed with this simple garlic-tarragon vinaigrette. Serve as a side dish with beef or lamb.

NET CARBS PER SERVING: *4 grams*

CARBOHYDRATES PER SERVING: *8.2 grams*

225 g green beans, trimmed
5 tablespoons olive oil
50 g finely chopped onion
1 garlic clove, finely chopped
2 tablespoons white wine
    vinegar

1 tablespoon chopped fresh
    tarragon leaves or 1½
    teaspoons crumbled dried
    tarragon
salt and pepper to taste

• Bring 2 litres of salted water to the boil in a large saucepan. Add the beans and cook for 5 to 6 minutes, or until tender. Drain the beans and refresh them under cold water to stop the cooking. Whisk together the olive oil, onion, garlic, vinegar, tarragon, salt and pepper.

Transfer the beans to a serving bowl. Pour the vinaigrette over them and toss well. Let the beans stand for 10 minutes. Serve immediately or store in an airtight container in the refrigerator for up to 1 day.

Serves 2

• Mangetout with Hazelnuts •

Flavoursome roasted nuts make a wonderful addition to sautéed vegetables. Hazelnuts, which are sometimes called filberts, are among our favourites.

> NET CARBS PER SERVING: 4 grams
>
> CARBOHYDRATES PER SERVING: 10.1 grams

75 g bacon lardons
25 g butter
225 g mangetout, washed

2 tablespoons hazelnuts, skinned
salt and pepper to taste

• Heat a large, heavy frying pan over a medium-high heat until hot. Sauté the bacon, stirring occasionally, for about 2 minutes, until browned. Remove the bacon from the frying pan and pour out the bacon fat. In the same frying pan heat the butter over a low heat until the foam subsides. Add the mangetout and cook until crisp-tender, about 1 minute.

Heat a small frying pan over a medium heat until hot. Add the hazelnuts and roast, shaking the frying pan occasionally, for 4 to 5 minutes, until golden and aromatic. Add the bacon, mangetout, salt and pepper, and sauté over a medium-high heat for 2 minutes. Serve immediately.

Serves 2 or 3

Variation: Substitute roasted walnuts for the hazelnuts and add 1 tablespoon of finely chopped fresh gingerroot and 1 tablespoon of soy sauce to the mangetout when adding the bacon.

• Green Beans with Anchovy Sauce •

Green beans are a great vehicle for this salty anchovy sauce. Serve as a side dish with Grilled Lemon and Rosemary Lamb (page 125).

NET CARBS PER SERVING: 3.2 grams

CARBOHYDRATES PER SERVING: 10 grams

450 g green beans, trimmed
    and washed
3 oil-packed anchovy fillets or
    1 tablespoon homemade
    Anchovy Paste (recipe on
    page 168) or prepared
    anchovy paste

25 g butter
100 ml chicken stock
1 tablespoon chopped basil for
    garnish

• Bring 2 litres of salted water to the boil in a large saucepan. Add the green beans and cook for 5 minutes. While the beans are cooking, combine the anchovy fillets or anchovy paste, butter and stock in a small saucepan and bring to a slow boil.

Drain the green beans and transfer them to a bowl. Pour the anchovy sauce over the beans, toss well, and garnish with the basil. Serve immediately.

Serves 2

• Green Bean, Smoked Mozzarella • and Tomato Salad

Beautiful, tasty and satisfying, this salad is hearty enough to serve as a starter.

> NET CARBS PER SERVING: *11 grams*
>
> CARBOHYDRATES PER SERVING: *17 grams*

225 g thin green beans
4 marinated artichoke hearts,
    drained and patted dry
2 plum tomatoes, thinly sliced
175 g smoked mozzarella
    cheese, cut into 0.5-cm
    slices

¼ cup walnut halves
Dressing:
3 tablespoons olive oil
2 teaspoons red wine vinegar
½ teaspoon Dijon mustard
½ teaspoon salt
¼ teaspoon pepper

• Cook the green beans in a large pot of lightly salted boiling water for 8 minutes, or until crisp-tender. Drain the beans and refresh them under cold water.

To assemble the salad: place two artichoke hearts in the centre of each plate. Encircle each artichoke heart with half the tomato slices. Arrange half the green beans and half the cheese slices around the artichokes. Sprinkle with half the walnuts.

For the dressing: Whisk the olive oil, vinegar, mustard, salt and pepper until well combined. Spoon the dressing over the salad.

Serves 2

• Sprouting Broccoli with Spicy • Sausage

The slightly bitter taste of sprouting broccoli is a perfect foil for spicy Italian sausage. The addition of balsamic vinegar adds a piquant tang. This dish makes a wonderful accompaniment to Grilled Marinated Lamb Chops (page 124) and can also serve as a light lunch on its own. The water that clings to the sprouting broccoli after it is washed should produce the right amount of liquid for cooking.

> NET CARBS PER SERVING: *8.9 grams*
>
> CARBOHYDRATES PER SERVING: *10.9 grams*

2 tablespoons olive oil
450 g hot Italian sausage, casings removed
2 cloves garlic, finely chopped
450 g sprouting broccoli, washed

1 tablespoon balsamic vinegar
1 teaspoon freshly ground black pepper
½ teaspoon dried hot red chilli pepper flakes
salt to taste

• Heat the oil in a large frying pan over a medium-high heat until hot but not smoking. Add the sausage and cook for 6 minutes, breaking up the lumps. Add the garlic and cook for another minute.

Turn the heat to low and add the sprouting broccoli and vinegar. (If the broccoli is too dry, add 1 teaspoon of water to the frying pan.) Cover and cook, stirring occasionally, for 7 minutes, or until the broccoli is tender. Stir in the pepper, hot chilli pepper flakes and salt. Serve immediately.

Serves 2

• Green Beans with Sun-Dried • Tomatoes and Goat's Cheese

The concentrated flavors of sun-dried tomatoes and goat's cheese, plus leeks and white wine, elevate green beans to an elegant side dish.

> NET CARBS PER SERVING: *8 grams*
>
> CARBOHYDRATES PER SERVING: *11 grams*

450 g green beans, trimmed and cut into 2.5-cm pieces

2 tablespoons extra virgin olive oil

2 leeks, white and 2.5-cm green, thinly sliced

2 garlic cloves, finely chopped

½ cup white wine

2 tablespoons oil-packed sun-dried tomatoes, drained and coarsely chopped

2 teaspoons chopped fresh thyme or ¾ teaspoon dried

salt and pepper

125 g soft goat's cheese, crumbled

• Cook the green beans in a large saucepan of lightly salted boiling water until crisp-tender, for about 5 minutes. Drain them and cool.

Heat the oil in a large frying pan over medium-high heat. Add the leeks and cook for 5 minutes, until softened. Add the garlic and cook for 1 minute more. Add the wine, tomatoes and thyme. Increase the heat to high and bring to the boil. Boil for 2 minutes until most of the wine evaporates. Mix in the green beans. Season to taste with salt and pepper. Transfer to a bowl, gently stirring in the goat's cheese. Serve immediately.

Serves 6

• Sautéed Spinach with Garlic • and Olive Oil

To this classic spinach dish we have added extra garlic and the earthy hint of nutmeg. This is the perfect accompaniment for Peppery Pork Chops (page 120).

NET CARBS PER SERVING: 4.3 grams

CARBOHYDRATES PER SERVING: 10.2 grams

3 tablespoons olive oil
4 large cloves garlic, sliced
300 g frozen leaf spinach,
    defrosted and drained
½ cube of chicken bouillon,
    crumbled

¼ teaspoon freshly grated
    nutmeg
salt and pepper to taste

• Heat the olive oil in a saucepan over a moderate heat until hot but not smoking. Add the garlic and cook for about 1 minute, until it begins to turn golden. Add the spinach and sprinkle with the crumbled chicken bouillon cube. Place a lid on the saucepan, leaving it slightly askew. Cook the spinach, stirring from time to time, until the moisture has evaporated, about 2–3 minutes. Turn off the heat and mix in the nutmeg, salt and pepper. Serve immediately.

Serves 2

• Puréed Avocado with Garlic •
and Tarragon

This purée has a vibrant green colour and creamy texture. It is a perfect accompaniment to prawn cocktail or cold salmon. Sometimes we like to use it in addition to mayonnaise for seafood and tuna salads. Remember this recipe when you have an avocado that has become too soft for other dishes.

> NET CARBS PER SERVING: 17.8 grams per 250 ml
>
> CARBOHYDRATES PER SERVING: 18.3 grams per 250 ml

1 ripe avocado (preferably Haas)
1 small clove garlic, finely chopped
1 tablespoon fresh lemon juice plus ½ teaspoon for sprinkling over the purée

1 tablespoon olive oil
3 tablespoons fresh tarragon leaves
salt and pepper to taste
2 tablespoons double cream

• Halve the avocado, remove the stone, and scoop the flesh into a food processor. Add the garlic, 1 tablespoon of lemon juice, oil, tarragon, salt and pepper. Purée the mixture for 30 seconds, or until smooth. With the motor running, add the cream and purée for another 15 seconds. Sprinkle the remaining lemon juice over the purée to prevent discolouration. Serve immediately or store in an airtight container in the refrigerator for up to 2 days.

Makes about 250 ml

• Roasted Peppers in Garlic Oil •

Roasting peppers is really extremely simple. Once the skin is charred, it pulls off easily, leaving the wonderfully sweet flesh. We sometimes chop roasted peppers and add them to chicken salad. Or we bathe the roasted peppers in garlic and oil, as in this recipe, and serve them as an accompaniment to grilled fish.

> NET CARBS PER SERVING: *3 grams*
> CARBOHYDRATES PER SERVING: *5.8 grams*

175 ml olive oil
2 cloves garlic, finely chopped

1 red pepper
1 green pepper

- Combine the oil and garlic in a bowl.

To roast on a gas burner: turn the flame to medium-high. Place the peppers directly on the flame and roast them, turning with tongs, for about 10 minutes, or until the skin is completely charred. (Alternately, you can roast the peppers in an oven pre-heated to 230°C/450°F, gas mark 8, turning them frequently with tongs, for about 20 minutes, or until the skin is completely charred.) Remove from the heat, place in a paper bag, and seal the bag by folding over the top. Allow the peppers to 'sweat' for 2 minutes.

Remove the peppers from the bag. Under running water pull the skin off the peppers. Remove the seeds and ribs, and add the roasted peppers to the garlic oil. Serve immediately.

Serves 2

· Vegetable Medley ·

The individual flavours of the vegetables remain distinct in this colourful medley. Serve with Garlic Dill Meatballs (page 121).

> NET CARBS PER SERVING: *4.2 grams*
>
> CARBOHYDRATES PER SERVING: *6 grams*

2 tablespoons olive oil
1 small onion, finely chopped
½ yellow pepper, diced
100 g diced courgettes
85 g peeled, seeded, and diced cucumber

50 ml chicken stock
2 cloves garlic, finely chopped
½ teaspoon cumin
¼ teaspoon dried oregano
salt and pepper to taste

- Heat the oil in a large frying pan over a medium-high heat until hot but not smoking. Add the onion, pepper, courgettes and cucumber, and sauté for 5 minutes, stirring occasionally. Add the chicken stock, garlic, cumin, oregano, salt and pepper. Bring to the boil, lower the heat, and simmer for 10 minutes, until the vegetables are tender. Serve immediately.

Serves 2

• Stir-Fried Vegetables with • Mustard Seeds and Balsamic Vinegar

This is a delicious and easy way to prepare a variety of vegetables you may have left over in your crisper. These are our favourite ingredients, but feel free to experiment. Other vegetables that work well in this stir-fry are snow peas, cauliflower, Brussels sprouts and mushrooms.

> NET CARBS PER SERVING: 6.8 grams
>
> CARBOHYDRATES PER SERVING: 8.3 grams

2 tablespoons olive oil
115 g broccoli florets
115 g runner or green beans, with the beans halved
1 tablespoon mustard seeds

2 large cloves garlic, finely chopped
½ teaspoon ground pepper
1 tablespoon balsamic vinegar
salt to taste

• Heat a large, heavy frying pan or wok over a medium-high heat for about 1 minute, until hot, and add the oil. Add the broccoli, beans, mustard seeds, garlic, pepper, vinegar and salt. Stir-fry the vegetables, stirring frequently, for about 10 minutes, or until tender. Serve hot or at room temperature.

Serves 2

• Stir-Fried Asparagus with Basil •

Asparagus is the premiere spring veggie. It is at its most tender and sweet early in the season. In this recipe, its sweetness is balanced with the peppery taste of basil.

> NET CARBS PER SERVING: 4.5 grams
>
> CARBOHYDRATES PER SERVING: 9 grams

2 tablespoons soy sauce
1 tablespoon water
1 packet sugar substitute (do not use Equal or aspartame; they lose their sweetness when heated)
1 tablespoon canola oil
1 jalapeño pepper, seeded and finely chopped
3 garlic cloves, finely chopped
675 g asparagus, lightly steamed and cut into 2.5-cm pieces
½ cup fresh basil leaves, thinly sliced

• In a small bowl, mix the soy sauce, water and sugar substitute. Heat the oil in a large frying pan over medium-high heat. Add the pepper and garlic, and cook for 30 seconds until the garlic is lightly browned. Stir in the asparagus, cook, whilst stirring, for 30 seconds. Add the soy sauce mixture and the basil. Cook until the basil just wilts.

Serves 4

• Spinach and Cheddar Casserole •

This rich, bubbly casserole pairs beautifully with simple grilled meat or chicken.

NET CARBS PER SERVING: *1.9 grams*

CARBOHYDRATES PER SERVING: *10.4 grams*

1 tablespoon olive oil
2 garlic cloves, finely chopped
900 g spinach, stemmed,
    washed and spun dry

2 tablespoons pine nuts
50 g grated Cheddar cheese

• Preheat the grill.

Heat the oil in a large frying pan over a medium heat until hot but not smoking. Add the garlic and cook for 1 minute, stirring occasionally. Add the spinach, cover, and cook for 5 minutes.

Transfer the spinach mixture to a small flameproof casserole and sprinkle with the pine nuts and Cheddar. Grill the casserole until the cheese is melted and lightly browned, about 2 minutes. Serve immediately.

Serves 2

• Sesame Broccoli •
Red Pepper and Spinach

This trio of vegetables is flavored Asian-style, with sesame, garlic, soy sauce and hot pepper. The mix makes a super-healthy year-round side dish that's delicious with beef, pork or lamb.

> NET CARBS PER SERVING: 3 grams
>
> CARBOHYDRATES PER SERVING: 5.5 grams

1 tablespoon sesame seeds

1 teaspoon canola oil

1 bunch broccoli, cut into 2.5-cm florets, stems peeled and cut into 5-cm x 0.5-cm strips

1 red pepper, cut into thin strips

1 garlic clove, crushed

1 bag (275 g) washed spinach

1 small hot red chilli or jalapeño pepper, seeded, finely chopped

1 tablespoon soy sauce

2 teaspoons sesame oil

• Toast the sesame seeds in a large non-stick frying pan over medium heat, stirring until the seeds are golden brown and fragrant. Transfer them to a small bowl.

Heat the oil over a medium heat in the same pan until it's hot. Add the broccoli and the red pepper. Cook until the broccoli is crisp-tender, which will be about 5 minutes. Add the garlic, spinach, jalapeño, soy sauce, and sesame oil. Mix them all together well. Cover and cook until the spinach is wilted, for about 2 minutes. Sprinkle the vegetables with toasted sesame seeds.

Serves 6

· Tomato-Cucumber Guacamole ·

This hearty salsa can be enjoyed as a side dish, a topping for salad greens or a savoury condiment for chicken, pork or burgers. For freshest flavour and brightest appearance, serve immediately after preparing.

> NET CARBS PER SERVING: *6 grams*
>
> CARBOHYDRATES PER SERVING: *11.5 grams*

1 pint cherry or grape tomatoes, halved, or 2 medium tomatoes, coarsely chopped

2 medium cucumbers (or 1 large seedless cucumber) peeled and coarsely chopped

2 Haas avocados, coarsely chopped

¼ cup red onion, chopped

1½ tablespoons lime juice

1 teaspoon freshly grated lime rind

½ teaspoon ground cumin

salt and pepper

• In a bowl, toss the tomatoes, cucumber, avocado, onion, lime juice, lime rind and cumin. Add the salt and pepper to taste.

Serves 8

Sauces

•

Sorrel Sauce

Red Pepper Purée

Anchovy Paste

Basil Pesto

Coriander-Lime Pesto

Mint-Cumin Pesto

Walnut and Blue Cheese Butter

Zesty Coriander Butter

Peanut Dipping Sauce

Cucumber-Dill Sauce

Creamy Celery Sauce

Horseradish Cream

Caper Tartar Sauce

Creamy Mushroom Sauce

Quick & Easy Hollandaise

• Sorrel Sauce •

Sorrel — a slightly sour herb that has grown wild for centuries throughout North America, Europe and Asia — is available in limited supply all year. It is worth seeking out, especially in the spring, when it is at its youngest and mildest. If you can't find sorrel, you can substitute rocket. Serve this elegant sauce with fish or chicken.

> NET CARBS: *11.9 grams per 250 ml (if using sorrel)*
> *6.2 grams per 250 ml (if using rocket)*
>
> CARBOHYDRATES: *13.6 grams per 250 ml (if using sorrel)*
> *7.9 grams per 250 ml (if using rocket)*

250 ml chicken stock
85 g trimmed sorrel, washed well
50 ml double cream

2 tablespoons chopped fresh dill
salt and pepper to taste

• Bring the chicken stock to the boil in a heavy saucepan over a medium-high heat. Turn the heat to low, add the sorrel, and simmer for 15 minutes, or until the sorrel is very wilted. Add the cream, dill, salt and pepper, and cook for 1 minute, or until the sauce is heated through (do not let it boil). Serve immediately.

Makes about 250 ml

• Red Pepper Purée •

This purée is always a big hit, and it is shamefully simple. Serve it with grilled or blackened tuna steaks. You can also thin the purée with some chicken stock to make a sprightly soup, which can be served warm or chilled.

> NET CARBS: 14.5 grams per 350 ml
>
> CARBOHYDRATES: 17.9 grams per 350 ml

1½ tablespoons olive oil
1 red pepper, chopped
1 roasted red pepper
    (procedure on page
    150), chopped, or 75 g
    chopped bottled roasted
    red pepper
2 cloves garlic, chopped

75 g chopped onion
2 tablespoons red wine
1½ teaspoons fresh lemon
    juice
1 tablespoon fresh tarragon
    leaves (optional)
salt and pepper to taste

• Heat the oil in a heavy frying pan over a medium heat until hot but not smoking. Add the peppers, garlic, onion and wine. Cover and cook for 6 minutes, stirring occasionally. (If the liquid begins to evaporate, add 1 to 2 tablespoons of water.) Remove from the heat and transfer to a food processor. Add the lemon juice, tarragon, salt and pepper, and purée for 30 seconds, or until smooth. Taste and adjust the seasoning. Serve immediately or store in an airtight container in the refrigerator for up to 3 days.

Makes about 350 ml

• Anchovy Paste •

Even though anchovy paste is available ready-made, we prefer to make it ourselves so we can control the saltiness. We keep it on hand for Caesar Dressing (page 186) or Green Beans with Anchovy Sauce (page 151).

> NET CARBS: 0.5 gram per 50 ml
>
> CARBOHYDRATES: 0.5 gram per 50 ml

one 55-g can oil-packed anchovies

1 tablespoon olive oil

1½ teaspoons grated lemon zest

• Gently rinse the anchovies in water, pat dry, and place in a food processor. Add the oil and lemon zest, and purée for 30 seconds, or until smooth. Scrape down the side and purée for another 5 seconds. (If the purée is too chunky, add a bit more oil and purée again.) Use immediately or store in an airtight container in the refrigerator for up to 1 week.

Makes 50 ml

• Basil Pesto •

This classic pesto is traditionally served on pasta — but not here!
Toss it with shredded cooked chicken for a lively chicken salad or
serve it as a condiment with grilled pork chops.

> NET CARBS: 9.3 grams per 175 ml
>
> CARBOHYDRATES: 9.8 grams per 175 ml

2 cloves garlic
100 g fresh basil leaves,
    washed and spun dry
3 tablespoons pine nuts

3 tablespoons grated Parmesan
    cheese
75 ml olive oil
salt and pepper to taste

• Place the garlic, basil leaves, pine nuts and Parmesan in a food processor and blend for a few seconds. Scrape down the side. With the motor running, add the oil in a steady stream and purée until smooth, about 1 minute. Transfer the pesto to a bowl and stir in the salt and pepper. Serve immediately or store, covered, in the refrigerator for up to 2 days.

Makes about 175 ml

• Coriander-Lime Pesto •

This pesto is divine when served with chicken or grilled fish.

> NET CARBS: 3.6 grams per 250 ml
>
> CARBOHYDRATES: 6 grams per 250 ml

75 g loosely packed fresh
   coriander leaves
1 clove garlic
½ tablespoon lime juice

40 g coarsely chopped walnuts
salt and pepper to taste
75 ml olive oil

• In a food processor, combine the coriander, garlic, lime juice, walnuts, salt and pepper. Process for 30 seconds and scrape down the side. With the motor running, add the oil in a slow stream and process for another 15 seconds, or until the pesto is smooth. Serve immediately or store in an airtight container in the refrigerator for up to 3 days or in the freezer for up to 2 weeks.

Makes about 250 ml

Hint:

For convenient future use, you can freeze the pesto in an ice-cube tray covered with cling film.

• Mint-Cumin Pesto •

Lively mint and aromatic cumin — an unusual team — pair up nicely in this flavoursome pesto. Serve it as a condiment with lamb.

NET CARBS: *10.1 grams per 250 ml*

CARBOHYDRATES: *12.5 grams per 250 ml*

75 g loosely packed mint
    leaves
1 clove garlic
1½ teaspoons fresh lime juice
40 g coarsely chopped
    walnuts, lightly toasted
    (see Hint on page 172)

1 teaspoon ground cumin
salt and pepper to taste
75 ml olive oil

• In a food processor, combine the mint, garlic, lime juice, walnuts, cumin, salt and pepper. Process for 30 seconds and scrape down the side. With the motor running, add the oil in a slow stream and process for another 15 seconds, or until smooth. Serve immediately or store in an airtight container in the refrigerator for up to 3 days or in the freezer for up to 2 weeks.

Makes about 250 ml

• Walnut and Blue Cheese Butter •

This rich butter can turn a simple cut of beef into an elegant and sophisticated dish. We also like to combine it with cauliflower florets and bake the mixture for a creative alternative to the traditional 'au gratin'.

NET CARBS: *1 gram per 100 g*

CARBOHYDRATES: *2.7 grams per 100 g*

55 g blue cheese, crumbled
20 g butter, softened
1 teaspoon finely chopped
　　fresh flat-leaf parsley
1 teaspoon finely chopped

fresh rosemary or thyme
1 tablespoon chopped walnuts,
　　toasted (see Hint)

• **Combine the blue cheese, butter, parsley, rosemary and walnuts in a glass or ceramic bowl and mix well. Serve the butter immediately or store it, covered, in the refrigerator for up to 3 days.**

Makes about 100 g

Hint: To toast nuts

Heat a heavy frying pan over a medium heat until hot. Add the nuts and cook, stirring constantly, for about 3 minutes, until very aromatic and beginning to turn brown. (Be careful that the nuts do not burn.) Remove from the heat. The toasted nuts can be served immediately, dusted lightly with salt, or stored in an airtight container for up to 1 week.

• Zesty Coriander Butter •

You can serve this wonderful butter on runner beans or use it to sauté broccoli. Try it instead of plain butter on the Sesame Soured Cream Muffins (page 193). Or liven up grilled chicken by topping it with a knob or two of the butter just before the chicken has finished cooking.

> NET CARBS: 4.2 grams per 50 g
>
> CARBOHYDRATES: 4.2 grams per 50 g

45 g butter, softened
1½ tablespoons chopped fresh coriander

1½ teaspoons grated lemon or lime zest
1 teaspoon fresh lemon or lime juice

- Combine the butter, coriander, zest and lemon juice in a bowl and mix well. Serve immediately or store in an airtight container in the refrigerator for up to 1 week.

Makes about 50 g

· Peanut Dipping Sauce ·

This peanut dipping sauce is so tasty and easy to make. Serve it with Coconut Chicken Satés with Coriander (page 105). You can also add a couple of tablespoons of dipping sauce to stir-fried vegetables for a distinctive Thai flavour.

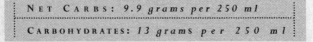

NET CARBS: *9.9 grams per 250 ml*

CARBOHYDRATES: *13 grams per 250 ml*

3 tablespoons peanut butter
1 tablespoon unsweetened
   coconut milk (optional)
1 tablespoon toasted sesame
   oil

100 ml water
1 tablespoon soy sauce
juice of ½ lime
1 small clove garlic
40 g chopped fresh coriander

• **Combine the peanut butter, coconut milk, if using, sesame oil, water, soy sauce, lime juice, garlic and coriander in a food processor and purée until smooth, about 1 minute. (If the sauce is too thick, add a bit more water.) Serve immediately or store, covered, in the refrigerator for up to 4 days.**

Makes about 250 ml

• Cucumber-Dill Sauce •

We serve this wonderfully versatile sauce with our Grilled Lemon
and Rosemary Lamb (page 125) or on top of a burger. You can
also whisk it with some olive oil for a quick salad dressing.

> **NET CARBS: 5.9 grams per 175 ml**
>
> **CARBOHYDRATES: 6.2 grams per 175 ml**

45 g diced cucumber
100 ml soured cream
1 teaspoon fresh lemon juice
1 tablespoon chopped fresh
    dill

1 teaspoon chopped fresh mint
1 small clove garlic, finely
    chopped
salt and pepper to taste

• **Combine the cucumber, soured cream, lemon juice, dill, mint,
garlic, salt and pepper in a glass or ceramic bowl and mix well.
Serve immediately or store in an airtight container in the
refrigerator for up to 2 days.**

Makes about 175 ml

• Creamy Celery Sauce •

Serve this cool, refreshing sauce with *Beef Burgers with Feta and Tomato* (page 136). It also works well as a dip for crudités.

NET CARBS: *6.5 grams per 175 ml*	
CARBOHYDRATES: *6.9 grams per 175 ml*	

100 ml soured cream
25 g finely chopped celery
1 teaspoon ground celery seeds

1½ teaspoons fresh lemon
    juice
salt and pepper to taste

• **Whisk together the soured cream, celery, celery seeds, lemon juice, salt and pepper in a bowl until the sauce is smooth. Serve immediately or store in an airtight container in the refrigerator for up to 4 days.**

Makes about 175 ml

• Horseradish Cream •

This versatile British sauce is served traditionally over thinly sliced steak or roast beef. It also makes an ideal accompaniment for cold Oven-Poached Salmon with Dill and Wine (page 97) or smoked fish.

> NET CARBS: 3.5 grams per 175 ml
>
> CARBOHYDRATES: 4.7 grams per 175 ml

75 ml double cream
1 teaspoon Dijon mustard
1½ tablespoons drained
    horseradish

1 tablespoon soured cream
salt and pepper to taste

• Blend the cream and mustard in a food processor or in a bowl with an electric mixer until the mixture forms soft peaks, about 1 minute. Whisk together the horseradish, soured cream, salt and pepper until smooth. Fold the mustard cream mixture into the horseradish mixture. Serve immediately or store in an airtight container in the refrigerator for up to 5 days.

Makes about 175 ml

· Caper Tartar Sauce ·

Tangy capers give a wonderful flavour and texture to this home-made tartar sauce. We like ours with a dash of hot sauce, but you can adjust the 'heat' according to your taste.

> NET CARBS: *2.9 grams per 175 ml*
>
> CARBOHYDRATES: *3.1 grams per 175 ml*

100 ml mayonnaise
1 tablespoon small capers or
    chopped large capers
1 teaspoon Dijon mustard
1 teaspoon drained
    horseradish

1½ teaspoons fresh lemon
    juice
1 teaspoon grated onion
salt and pepper to taste
dash of hot chilli pepper sauce
    (optional)

• In a bowl, whisk together the mayonnaise, capers, mustard, horseradish, lemon juice, onion, salt, pepper and hot chilli pepper sauce, if using, until smooth. Serve immediately or store in an airtight container in the refrigerator for up to 5 days.

Makes about 175 ml

• Creamy Mushroom Sauce •

This versatile mushroom sauce makes a great flavour enhancer for simple grilled steaks and chops as well as for Garlic Dill Meatballs (page 121).

> NET CARBS: *3 grams per 250 ml*
>
> CARBOHYDRATES: *8.2 grams per 250 ml*

15 g butter
225 g button mushrooms, finely chopped
100 ml chicken stock

2 tablespoons double cream
1 tablespoon soured cream
salt and pepper to taste
nutmeg to taste

• Heat the butter in a frying pan over a medium heat until the foam subsides. Add the mushrooms and cook for 5 minutes, stirring frequently. Add the chicken stock and double cream, and cook for 2 minutes. Remove from the heat and stir in the soured cream, salt, pepper and nutmeg. Serve immediately or store, covered, in the refrigerator for up to 1 day.

Makes about 250 ml

• Quick & Easy Hollandaise •

This blender version of the classic sauce is easy and delicious.
Serve it with Eggs Benedict with Spinach (page 31) or steamed
asparagus.

> NET CARBS: *1.3 grams per 100 ml*
>
> CARBOHYDRATES: *1.3 grams per 100 ml*

75 g butter
2 egg yolks
1 tablespoon fresh lemon juice

salt to taste
cayenne pepper to taste
nutmeg to taste (optional)

• Heat the butter in a saucepan over a low heat until gently
bubbling. Meanwhile, place the egg yolks in a blender or food
processor and blend for a few seconds. With the motor running,
add the lemon juice, salt, cayenne and nutmeg, if using. Slowly
add the melted butter in a thin stream and blend for 10 seconds,
or until thickened and smooth.

Makes about 100 ml

Dressings

•

Quick & Easy Salad Dressing
Shallot Orange Vinaigrette
Mustard Walnut Vinaigrette
Caesar Dressing
Smoked Salmon Dressing

• Quick & Easy Salad Dressing •

Bottled salad dressings often contain sugar or corn syrup, which boost the carbohydrate grams. You can make your own delicious dressing with some basic ingredients that you probably have in your cupboards.

NET CARBS: *5.4 grams per 100 ml*

CARBOHYDRATES: *5.4 grams per 100 ml*

2 oil-packed anchovy fillets
3 tablespoons olive oil
1½ tablespoons good-quality
    vinegar (such as wine,
    balsamic or sherry)

1 tablespoon Dijon mustard
salt and pepper to taste

• Mash the anchovy fillets with a fork. Place in a small jar that has a tight-fitting lid. Add the oil, vinegar, mustard, salt and pepper. Cover with the lid and shake vigorously until well blended, about 15 to 30 seconds. Serve immediately or store in the refrigerator, covered, for up to 4 days. Shake the dressing before serving.

Makes about 100 ml

· Shallot Orange Vinaigrette ·

Homemade salad dressings taste so much better than the bottled versions. This tangy, slightly sweet vinaigrette can also be used as a marinade for beef, pork or lamb.

> **NET CARBS:** *12.9 grams per 250 ml*
>
> **CARBOHYDRATES:** *13.1 grams per 250 ml*

2 tablespoons balsamic vinegar

2 tablespoons red wine vinegar

2 teaspoons Worcestershire sauce

2 teaspoons Dijon mustard

1 tablespoon lime juice

1 tablespoon finely chopped shallots

1 teaspoon grated orange zest

1 teaspoon fresh orange juice

salt and pepper to taste

175 ml olive oil

• In a food processor, combine the balsamic vinegar, red wine vinegar, Worcestershire sauce, mustard, lime juice, shallots, zest, orange juice, salt and pepper, and blend for 30 seconds. With the motor running, add the oil in a slow stream and blend for another 20 seconds, or until the vinaigrette is smooth. Use immediately or store in an airtight container in the refrigerator for up to 1 week.

Makes about 250 ml

• Mustard Walnut Vinaigrette •

A generous measure of mustard gives this vinaigrette a pungent flavour. It is a tasty alternative to mayonnaise-based dressings.

> NET CARBS: 4.5 grams per 175 ml
>
> CARBOHYDRATES: 4.5 grams per 175 ml

1½ tablespoons Dijon mustard
3 tablespoons red wine vinegar
1 small clove garlic
½ teaspoon salt
½ teaspoon freshly ground pepper
100 ml olive oil
1 tablespoon walnut oil

• In a food processor or blender, combine the mustard, vinegar, garlic, salt and pepper, and blend for 30 seconds. With the motor running, add the oils in a slow stream and blend for another 10 seconds, or until the vinaigrette is smooth. Use immediately or store in an airtight container in the refrigerator for up to 1 week.

Makes about 175 ml

• Caesar Dressing •

Because raw eggs have fallen out of favour due to the risks associated with salmonella, we have created a version of this classic dressing with a hard-boiled egg. The dressing will separate because the hard-cooked egg cannot 'hold' the oil. If you prepare the dressing ahead of time, be sure to reblend it before serving.

> NET CARBS: 4.8 grams per 175 ml
>
> CARBOHYDRATES: 4.9 grams per 175 ml

1 hard-boiled egg, peeled
2 small cloves garlic
1½ tablespoons Anchovy Paste
  (page 168)
1 teaspoon fresh lemon juice
1 tablespoon Worcestershire
  sauce

½ teaspoon Dijon mustard
2 tablespoons olive oil
2 tablespoons grated Parmesan
  cheese

• Place the egg, garlic, anchovy paste, lemon juice, Worcestershire sauce and mustard in a food processor and purée for 30 seconds, or until smooth. With the motor running, add the oil in a slow stream and then the Parmesan and purée for another 30 seconds, or until smooth. Use immediately or store in an airtight container in the refrigerator for up to 3 days. Reblend the dressing before serving.

Makes about 175 ml

• Smoked Salmon Dressing •

This unusual dressing is great on mixed salad greens. It is also delicious when served as an accompaniment to steamed asparagus or as a dip for crudités.

> **NET CARBS:** *8.4 grams per 250 ml*
>
> **CARBOHYDRATES:** *8.5 grams per 250 ml*

50 ml soured cream
100 ml mayonnaise
45 g smoked salmon, thinly
    sliced
2 teaspoons white wine
    vinegar

3 teaspoons fresh lemon juice
2 tablespoons chopped spring
    onions (white part only)

• Combine the soured cream, mayonnaise, salmon, vinegar, lemon juice and spring onions in a food processor and purée for 1 minute, or until smooth. Serve immediately or store in an airtight container in the refrigerator for up to 2 days.

Makes about 250 ml

Breads

•

Cheddar Cheese Bread
Bacon Pepper Bread
Sesame Soured Cream Muffins
Butter Rum Muffins

• Cheddar Cheese Bread •

Infused with mellow Cheddar, this bread is rich and satisfying.

NET CARBS: 11.6 grams per loaf	
CARBOHYDRATES: 18 grams per loaf	

butter for greasing the loaf tin
60 g soya flour (available at
    natural-food stores)
4 tablespoons whey protein
    (available at natural-
    food stores)

2 large eggs
½ teaspoon baking powder
2 tablespoons soured cream
2 tablespoons olive oil
grated Cheddar cheese

• Preheat the oven to 190°C/375°F, gas mark 5. Generously butter a loaf tin, 20 by 10 by 6-cm.

Combine the soya flour, whey, eggs, baking powder, soured cream and oil in a bowl and mix well. Fold in half of the Cheddar. Pour the batter into the tin and sprinkle the remaining Cheddar on top. Bake for 25 minutes, or until a skewer inserted in the middle comes out clean. Serve immediately or store, wrapped well in cling film, in the refrigerator for up to 2 days or in the freezer for up to 1 month.

Makes 1 loaf

• Bacon Pepper Bread •

Serve this appetizing bread with eggs for breakfast or with a big salad for a light lunch.

> NET CARBS: *12.4 grams per loaf*
> CARBOHYDRATES: *18.8 grams per loaf*

butter for greasing the loaf tin
60 g soya flour (available at natural-food stores)
4 tablespoons whey protein (available at natural-food stores)
2 large eggs

½ teaspoon baking powder
2 tablespoons soured cream
½ teaspoon freshly ground pepper
3 rashers bacon, cooked and crumbled

• Preheat the oven to 190°C/375°F, gas mark 5. Generously butter a loaf tin, 20 by 10 by 6-cm.

Combine the soya flour, whey, eggs, baking powder, soured cream and pepper in a bowl and mix well. Fold in half of the bacon bits. Pour the batter into the prepared tin and sprinkle the remaining bacon on top. Bake for 25 minutes, or until a skewer inserted in the middle comes out clean. Serve immediately or store, wrapped well in cling film, in the refrigerator for up to 2 days or in the freezer for up to 1 month.

Makes 1 loaf

• Sesame Soured Cream Muffins •

Go ahead — spread butter, cream cheese or pâté on these savoury muffins. You'll never miss the old white bread. They make a great accompaniment for soup or a salad.

> NET CARBS: *2.6 grams per muffin*
>
> CARBOHYDRATES: *3.8 grams per muffin*

45 g tofu or soya flour
    (available at natural-
    food stores)
25 g ground sesame seeds (see
    Hint on page 190)

3 tablespoons soured cream
25 g butter, melted
½ teaspoon baking powder
2 large eggs, lightly beaten

● Preheat the oven to 180°C/350°F, gas mark 4. Generously butter four muffin tins.

Combine the flour, sesame seeds, soured cream, melted butter, baking powder and eggs in a food processor and process for 2 to 3 minutes, or until smooth. Divide the batter evenly among the 4 muffin tins, filling each about half full. Fill the empty muffin tins with water. Bake for 20 to 25 minutes, or until a skewer inserted in the middle comes out clean. Let the muffins cool in the tins for 5 minutes, then turn them out on to a rack to cool completely.

Makes 4 muffins

• Butter Rum Muffins •

You'll hardly feel deprived when you sit down to a breakfast of these delicious muffins spread with butter and a hot cup of coffee (decaf, of course) with double cream.

> NET CARBS: 2.6 grams per muffin
>
> CARBOHYDRATES: 3.8 grams per muffin

45 g tofu or soya flour (available at natural-food stores)

25 g ground sesame seeds

3 tablespoons whey protein (available at some natural-food stores)

2 large eggs, lightly beaten

3 tablespoons soured cream

15 g butter, softened

1 teaspoon rum

1½ g Splenda (do not use Equal or aspartame; they lose their sweetness when heated)

½ teaspoon vanilla extract

½ teaspoon baking powder

• Preheat the oven to 180°C/350°F, gas mark 4. Generously butter four 100-ml muffin tins.

Combine the flour, sesame seeds, whey protein, eggs, soured cream, butter, rum, sugar substitute, vanilla extract and baking powder in a food processor and process for 2 to 3 minutes, or until smooth. Divide the batter evenly among the 4 muffin tins, filling each about half full, and fill empty muffin tins with water. Bake for 20 to 25 minutes, or until a a skewer inserted in the middle comes out clean. Let the muffins cool in the tins for 5 minutes, then turn them out on to a rack to cool completely.

Variation: For luscious homemade blueberry muffins, add 40 g blueberries (5.1 grams carbohydrate) to the batter.

Makes 4 muffins

Desserts

•

Zabaglione

Swedish Cream

Coconut Custard Pudding

Chocolate Butter Cream

Hazelnut Torte

Crustless Cheesecake

Coconut Cookies

Shortcake Veronique with a Kiss of Rum

Dr Atkins' Quick and Easy Dessert

· Zabaglione ·

This luxurious custard is fused with rich marsala wine and complemented by fresh berries. It is the perfect ending for a dinner or a brunch. Enjoy!

> NET CARBS PER SERVING: *4.7 grams*
>
> CARBOHYDRATES PER SERVING: *5.3 grams*

4 egg yolks
1½ g Splenda (do not use
    Equal or aspartame; they
    lose their sweetness when
    heated)
50 ml dry Marsala wine

40 g blueberries
2 large ripe strawberries
2 sprigs fresh mint leaves,
    washed and dried for
    garnish

• Combine the egg yolks, Splenda and Marsala in a food processor and blend for about 15 seconds. Pour the mixture into the top of a double boiler or a bowl set over a pan of gently simmering water and whisk constantly for about 5 minutes, until it thickens to the consistency of whipped cream. Pour into 2 small bowls or ramekins. Garnish each with half of the blueberries, a strawberry and a sprig of mint leaves. Serve or chill. The custard can be chilled and served for up to 3 days.

Serves 2

• Swedish Cream •

This is so simple to prepare, yet tastes wonderfully decadent!

NET CARBS PER SERVING: 4.35 grams

CARBOHYDRATES PER SERVING: 4.35 grams

100 ml double cream
2½ teaspoons unflavoured
    gelatin
1½ g Splenda (do not use
    Equal or aspartame; they
    lose their sweetness when
    heated)

½ teaspoon vanilla extract
100 ml soured cream

• Combine half of the double cream and the gelatin in a small saucepan and cook over a very low heat, whisking constantly, for 1 to 2 minutes, until the gelatin is dissolved. Slowly add the remaining double cream, whisking constantly. Add the Splenda and vanilla extract, and cook for 10 minutes, whisking frequently. Cool to room temperature. Whisk in the soured cream until the cream is smooth. Serve at room temperature or chilled.

Makes about 250 ml

Variation: For a more piquant taste, add ½ teaspoon of grated lemon zest to the cream when adding the soured cream.

· Coconut Custard Pudding ·

Rich and creamy, this coconut pudding has delicious butter-scotch undertones.

> **NET CARBS PER SERVING:** *8.6 grams*
>
> **CARBOHYDRATES PER SERVING:** *8.6 grams*

one 400 ml can unsweetened
    coconut milk
100 ml double cream
1 tablespoon butterscotch
    extract
3 egg yolks

3 g Splenda (do not use Equal
    or aspartame; they lose
    their sweetness when
    heated) (see Note)

● Bring the coconut milk and double cream to the boil in a saucepan, reduce turn the heat to very low.

Meanwhile, whisk together the butterscotch extract, egg yolks and sugar substitute in a bowl.

Whisk the egg mixture into the cream mixture, a little at a time, until incorporated. Simmer over a very low heat, stirring constantly, for 5 minutes. Transfer the pan to a large bowl or sink filled with cold water and let cool for 5 minutes. Serve the pudding at room temperature or chilled.

Serves 2

Note: If you combine more than one sweetner, they have a synergistic effect and less is needed. Use 2 grams instead of 3.

• Chocolate Butter Cream •

This velvety chocolate cream tastes great either on its own, served in individual glass bowls, or as an accompaniment to Hazelnut Torte (page 201).

> NET CARBS: 4.4 grams per 250 ml
>
> CARBOHYDRATES: 4.4 grams per 250 ml

4 large egg yolks
2 tablespoons Cognac
½ teaspoon vanilla extract
1 tablespoon shaved
 unsweetened dark
 chocolate
115 g unsalted butter,
 softened

1 g Splenda (do not use Equal
 or aspartame; they lose
 their sweetness when
 heated)

• Beat the egg yolks, Cognac, vanilla extract, chocolate, butter and Splenda in a large bowl with an electric mixer for 2 minutes. Place the mixture in the top of a double boiler or in a bowl set over a pan of gently simmering water and cook it for 7 minutes, stirring constantly. Remove from the heat, let cool to room temperature, and serve.

Makes about 250 ml or 2 servings

• Hazelnut Torte •

This baked hazelnut torte has a rich flavour and a wonderful aroma. Serve with whipped cream or Chocolate Butter Cream (page 200).

> NET CARBS PER SERVING: 3.8–5.3 grams
>
> CARBOHYDRATES PER SERVING: 5.5–7.4 grams

butter for greasing the cake tin
75 g ground hazelnuts
1 tablespoon whey protein (available at natural-food stores)
2 large eggs

1 tablespoon soured cream
1 Splenda (do not use Equal or aspartame; they lose their sweetness when heated)
½ tablespoon baking powder

• Preheat the oven to 180°C/350°F, gas mark 4.

Generously butter an 20-cm round cake tin and sprinkle 2 tablespoons of hazelnuts over the bottom.

Combine the remaining hazelnuts, whey protein, eggs, soured cream, Splenda and baking powder in a large bowl. Using an electric mixer, blend at medium-high speed for about 2 minutes, until fluffy. Pour the batter into the prepared tin. Bake for 25 minutes, or until a skewer comes out clean. Cool to room temperature and serve.

Serves 3 or 4

• Crustless Cheesecake •

There's no need to give up rich, luscious desserts while you're on the Atkins diet. Here's a sublime crustless cheesecake that is sure to delight sweet teeth everywhere.

> NET CARBS PER SERVING: 2.4 grams
>
> CARBOHYDRATES PER SERVING: 2.6 grams

350 g cream cheese, softened
3 g Splenda (see Note)
1 teaspoon vanilla extract
250 ml double cream

85 g fresh strawberries, quartered (optional / 5.2 grams of carbohydrate)

• Combine the cream cheese, sugar substitute and vanilla extract in a bowl and mix well. Beat the double cream in a bowl until it forms soft peaks. Fold the whipped cream into the cream cheese mixture.

Transfer the mixture to a large glass bowl and chill, covered with cling film, for at least 25 minutes. Top with the berries, if using. Serve immediately or store, covered with cling film, in the refrigerator for up to 2 days.

Serves 8

Note: If you use a combination of artificial sweeteners, they have a synergistic effect. Therefore, less is needed. Use 2 grams instead of 3.

• Coconut Cookies •

Yes, you can indulge in fresh-baked biscuits! These nutty clusters are a marvellous treat. When baking these cookies, be sure to leave plenty of room around them so they can spread out.

NET CARBS: *0.1 gram per cookie*

CARBOHYDRATES: *0.9 grams per cookie*

butter for greasing the baking sheet
85 g Atkins Bake Mix*
25 g unsweetened desiccated coconut
45 g coarsely chopped hazelnuts
2 egg whites

2 tablespoons fizzy mineral water
115 g butter, softened
2 g different sugar substitute or 3 g Splenda (do not use Equal or aspartame; they lose their sweetness when heated) (see Note)

● Preheat the oven to 190°C/375°F, gas mark 5.
Generously butter a baking sheet.
Combine the bake mix, coconut, hazelnuts, egg whites, mineral water, butter and sugar substitute in a bowl and mix well. Drop the batter by rounded tablespoons on to the prepared baking sheet (you will have about 20). Bake for 20 minutes, or until lightly golden. Remove from the oven and cool slightly. Serve immediately or store in an airtight container for up to 1 week.

Makes about 20 cookies

Note: We suggest using a combination of sugar substitutes because when different types are used together, they have a synergistic effect. Therefore, less is needed.

* Available from www.atkinscenter.com

• Shortcake Veronique •
with a Kiss of Rum

No one will believe that this dessert is part of a diet. The rum adds a depth of flavour that is perfectly complemented by the fresh berries.

> NET CARBS PER SERVING: *7.1 grams*
>
> CARBOHYDRATES PER SERVING: *8.5 grams*

2 butter rum muffins (recipe on page 194), halved

2 teaspoons rum (do not substitute liqueurs, because they are high in sugar)

100 ml double cream

1 g Splenda

2 large strawberries, halved

• **Sprinkle the muffin halves with the rum. Combine the cream and Splenda in a bowl and beat until soft peaks form. Divide the whipped cream among the muffin halves. Place a strawberry half in the centre of each shortcake half. Serve immediately.**

Serves 2

• Dr Atkins's Quick • & Easy Dessert

When I don't have time to make a dessert, I will invariably find Dr Atkins in the kitchen improvising a sweet finale. This is one of his best concoctions.

> NET CARBS PER SERVING: *4.8 grams*
>
> CARBOHYDRATES PER SERVING: *6 grams*

2 coconut cookies (recipe on
    page 203) or 25 g
    unsweetened desiccated
    coconut
50 ml soured cream
50 ml double cream

2 large strawberries, sliced
2 g different sugar substitutes
    or 3 g of Splenda (see
    Note)*
a dash of rum or Cognac

• Divide the cookies, crumbled, or the coconut between 2 small serving bowls. Top each serving with half of the soured cream, half of the double cream, half of the strawberries, half of the Splenda and a sprinkling of rum. Serve immediately.

Serves 2

Note: We suggest using a combination of artificial sweeteners because when different types are used together, they have a synergistic effect. Therefore, less is needed.

* Although most published scientific studies have proclaimed aspartame (NutraSweet, Equal) to be safe, clinical experience has often indicated otherwise. Headaches, irritability and failure to lose weight or to control blood glucose have all been reported, as well as cross reactions in those who cannot tolerate monosodium glutamate (MSG). Consult with your doctor if you have any concern about your use of aspartame. The best advice may be to use it sparingly, preferably blending it with other sweeteners. Remember, too, that aspartame loses its sweetness when heated.

PROTEINS

BEEF

ALL CHEESES*

(AGED)

Blue cheeses
Brie
Camembert
Cheddar
Feta
Fontina
Goat's cheese
Gouda
Gruyère
Havarti (Danish)
Monterey Jack
Mozzarella
Münster (German)
Parmigiano
Pecorino
Provolone
Romano

(FRESH)

Cottage
Cream
Goat's
Mascarpone
Ricotta

CHICKEN
DUCK
EGGS
ALL FISH
(INCLUDING CANNED)

Anchovy
Bass
Bluefish
Catfish
Cod
Flounder
Haddock
Monk
Red snapper
Salmon
Sardines
Sole
Swordfish
Trout
Tuna
Whitefish

SHELLFISH

Clams
Crab
Crayfish
Lobster
Mussels
Oysters
Prawns
Scallops
Squid

* For cheeses you should avoid,
see Hidden Carbohydrates on
pages 20–21.

GAME BIRDS
LAMB
MILK PRODUCTS
  Butter
  Cream
  Soured cream
  Whipped cream

PORK
RABBIT
TURKEY
VEAL
VENISON

SALAD
VEGETABLES
AND GREENS

  Alfalfa sprouts
  Bean sprouts
  Bok choy (pak choi)
  Cabbage
  Celery
  Chicory
  Chinese cabbage
  Chives
  Cucumber
  Endive
  Escarole
  Fennel
  Jicama
  Kale
  Leeks
  Lettuce
  Mushrooms
  Mustard greens
  Okra
  Peppers

Radishes
Rocket
Sorrel
Spinach
Swiss chard
Watercress

OTHER
VEGETABLES LOW IN
CARBOHYDRATES

  Artichoke
  Aubergine
  Asparagus
  Avocado
  Broccoli
  Brussels sprouts
  Cauliflower
  Courgettes
  Kohlrabi
  Mangetout
  Onions
  Plantains
  Pumpkin
  Rhubarb
  Sauerkraut
  Spaghetti squash
  Spring onions
  Sprouting Broccoli
  String/green beans
  Turnips
  Water chestnuts

HERBS
  Basil
  Bay leaf
  Chervil
  Chives

Coriander
Dill
Lemongrass
Marjoram
Mint
Oregano
Parsley
Rosemary
Sage
Tarragon
Thyme

NUTS AND SEEDS

Almonds
Brazil nuts
Coconut (fresh)
Filberts (hazelnuts)
Macadamias
Pecans
Pine nuts
Pumpkin seeds
Sesame seeds
Sunflower seeds
Walnuts

FATS AND OILS
(Cold-pressed oils are preferred.)

Animal fat
Butter
Mayonnaise
Olive oil
Rapeseed oil
Safflower oil
Sesame oil
Soybean oil
Sunflower oil
Walnut oil

FLOUR AND COATINGS

Atkins Bake Mix
Pork rinds
Soya flour
Tofu flour
Whey protein

SUGAR SUBSTITUTES

Splenda
Stevia

Each person must determine the sweeteners that agree with him or her.* The most efficient way to use sweeteners is to use more than one type together because sweeteners create a synergistic effect. You should experiment with combinations until you discover your favourite and the amount to use for desired sweetness.

*Although most published scientific studies have proclaimed aspartame (NutraSweet, Equal) to be safe, clinical experience has often indicated otherwise. Headaches, irritability and failure to lose weight or to control blood glucose have all been reported, as well as cross reactions in those who cannot tolerate monosodium glutamate (MSG). Consult with your doctor if you have any concern about your use of aspartame. The best advice may be to use it sparingly, preferably blending it with other sweeteners. Remember, too, that aspartame loses its sweetness when heated.

Looking for a Controlled Carbohydrate Connection?

Right now there are exciting new low-carbohydrate foods and baking products available to you. Contact us for more information and make this *quick* and *easy* diet even quicker and easier.

Also, if you are interested in further information about:

- Specially formulated nutritional supplements for diet and health
- Dr Atkins' national monthly newsletter
- Atkins Diet vacation cruises
- Controlled carbohydrate food products

Visit our Website:

www.atkinscenter.com

Or write to:

THE ATKINS CENTER FOR COMPLEMENTARY MEDICINE
152 EAST 55TH STREET
NEW YORK, NY 10022

• Acknowledgments •

A VERY SPECIAL THANKS TO . . .

My sister, Valentina Zimbalkin, whose culinary talents I have always admired and secretly envied.

Our friend Anya Senoret, whose creativity extends from designing beautiful clothes to creating wonderful dishes.

Nena, who was visiting from Croatia.

My niece and nephew, Tina and Michael (eight and ten years old), who were my 'official tasters' and whose verdicts of 'cool' and 'awesome' were very encouraging.

My former roommate, Stella Siu, who gave me some wonderful pointers.

Kathleen Duffy Freud, Bettina Newman and Michael Cohn for their expertise and assistance.

My editors at Simon & Schuster, Fred Hills and Sydny Miner, for their faith and support under daunting deadlines.

Erika Sommer, my coauthor, without whom this book would not have been born.

Nancy Hancock, last but not least, who convinced Simon & Schuster that this book 'needed to be!'

ABOUT THE AUTHORS

ROBERT C. ATKINS, MD, is the founder and medical director of the Atkins Center for Complementary Medicine. A 1951 graduate of the University of Michigan, he received his medical degree from Cornell University Medical School in 1955, and went on to specialize in cardiology. He has been a practising physician for over thirty years and is the author of several books. As a leader in the areas of natural medicine and nutritional pharmacology, he has built an international reputation. He is the recipient of the World Organization of Alternative Medicine's Recognition of Achievement Award and was the US National Health Federation's Man of the Year. His many media appearances, where he has discussed diet and health, include *Larry King Live*, *Oprah*, *CBS This Morning*, and *CNBC*, among others. Many magazine and newspaper articles have featured his work, and he also has a nationally syndicated radio show in America. He lives in New York City with his wife, Veronica.

VERONICA ATKINS was born in Russia and narrowly escaped the Nazi onslaught during World War II by fleeing to live with her great-aunt in Vienna. In the years since, she has lived in seven countries and become fluent in as many languages. Her far-flung travels have given her an extensive knowledge of international cuisine. Music has also played an important role in her life. She began singing in Europe at a young age and performed professionally as an opera singer from 1963 to 1976. Today she is actively involved in Dr Atkins' work at The Atkins Center for Complementary Medicine. She serves on the board of directors of the Foundation for the Advancement of Innovative Medicine Education group. Her current stage is the kitchen, where she actively creates and develops delicious low-carbohydrate recipes.

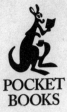

POCKET
BOOKS

DR ATKINS
VITA-NUTRIENT SOLUTION
Your Complete Guide to Natural Health
Dr Robert Atkins

Author of the bestselling
Dr Atkins New Diet Revolution

Long a champion of complementary medicine
and nutritional therapy, Dr Robert Atkins
presents the scientific basis of the use of vitamins,
minerals, amino acids, herbs, and hormones in the
treatment and prevention of most of the chronic
illnesses that plague us today.

Best of all, Dr Atkins shows consumers how to
create a personalised programme to help them
harness the body's ability to heal itself, rather
than resorting to conventional drugs and invasive
procedures. *The Vita-Nutrient Solution* address the
true cause of disease instead of temporarily
alleviating symptoms, promoting longer-lasting
and more effective healing.

PRICE £8.99
ISBN 0 7434 2997 4